The Pregnancy-After-30 Workbook

The Pregnancy-After-30 Workbook

A Program for Safe Childbearing—No Matter What Your Age

Edited by

Gail Sforza Brewer

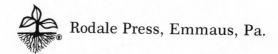 Rodale Press, Emmaus, Pa.

Library of Congress Cataloging in Publication Data
Main entry under title:

The Pregnancy-after-30 workbook.

Bibliography: p.
Includes index.
1. Pregnancy in middle age. 2. Childbirth in middle age.   I. Brewer, Gail Sforza.
RG556.6.P73   618.2'4   78-15008
ISBN 0-87857-215-5

Printed in the United States of America on recycled paper, containing a high percentage of de-inked fiber.

4 6 8 10 9 7 5 3

Contents

For My Mother

Acknowledgments

Some individuals whose assistance helped make this book possible are: Nancy Devore, C.N.M. of Albert Einstein Hospital, Bronx, New York and Lonnie Holtzman, C.N.M. of Maternity Center Associates in Englewood Cliffs, New Jersey, who arranged for our photographers to be present during the births depicted; and Charles Gerras, the editor on the project, whose patience and goodwill have turned most of the work on this book into pleasure.

To Marge and Jay Hathaway goes my deepest appreciation; without their early dedication to improved health for all mothers and babies, the contributors to this book would never have become acquainted.

G.S.B.
Croton-on-Hudson, N.Y.
March 8, 1978

Photograph credits

Vince Basile, pages viii, ix, 50, 52, 56, 61, 62, 70, 96, 97, 107, 109, 110, 111, 141

Steve Dalber, pages viii, ix, 110, 111, 134, 138, 159, 162

Rodger Parsons, pages 154, 155

John Crockett, page 78

Allan Tannenbaum, page 152

Geisinger Medical Center, Photography Department, page 46

Line drawings

by Pam and Walter Carroll

Many people generously shared their pregnancies, births, and family life with the contributors to this book. Special thanks to those pictured here. Their comments appear in the margins throughout the book, comparing their experiences with the material presented by the "experts." Each pregnancy affects the lives of the people involved in a unique way. Whether this is your first pregnancy or your fifth, these parents' reactions provide additional insight into childbearing after 30.

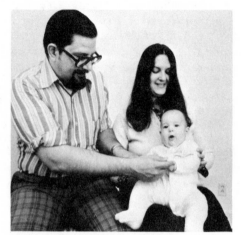

Susan and Frank Prezelski

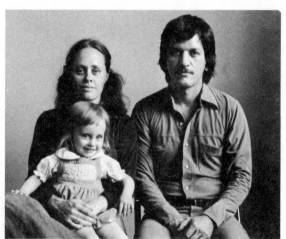

Jean and Steve Dalber

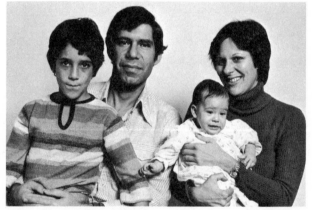

Mattie and Dave Perelman

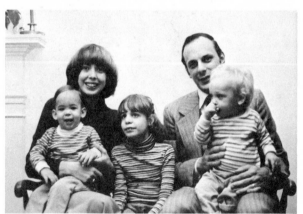

Judy and Dolf Beil

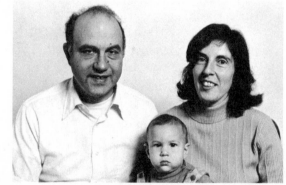

Elaine and Ed Gilbert

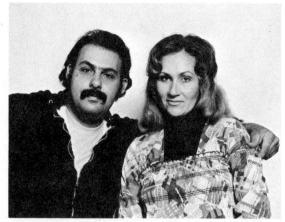

Karen and Gary Pecora

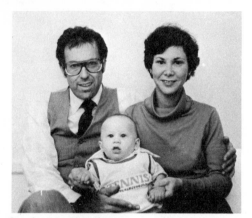

Carol and Al Tucker

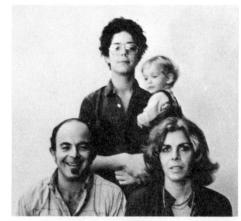

Edie and Norm Grossman

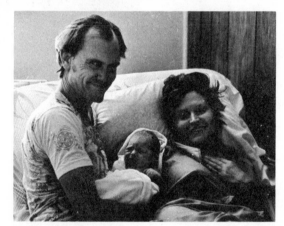

Chris and Clint Allmon

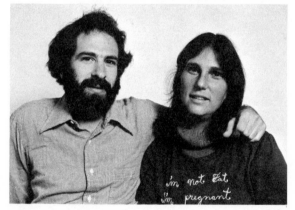

Karen and Mike Henes

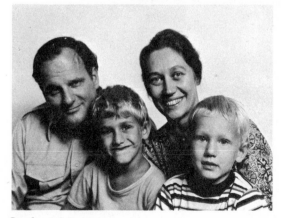

Sandy and Joe Jamong

Editor's Foreword

A phone call three years ago first alerted me to the idea that childbearing is "different" for women past the age of 30.

The caller was a 39-year-old expectant mother who had read a local newspaper's story about my series of childbirth education classes. She was worried. She had been told that having a baby at her time of life was going to be a life-threatening experience she would be lucky to survive—and that there was nothing she could do about it except to wait and see what kind of hand fate would deal her.

Edie Grossman was the caller. She holds a doctorate in Spanish, is a published translator, and chairman of the Humanities Division at Dominican College in Rockland County, New York. She is not the kind of person to leave her baby's future and her own to fate and a negative prognosis.

Instead, as she recounts here, she set out to make her pregnancy as healthful as possible—on her own terms!

"I gave birth to my first child on December 21, 1975. I was 39 years old and nervous:

- I had been told by a New York City birth center that I was statistically a "high risk" and could not have my baby there.
- The first obstetrician I consulted talked matter-of-factly about having to do a Cesarean section because of my age.
- The books I read subscribed to the conventional wisdom that first labors are long, painful, and arduous—especially if the woman is older.
- The only childbirth preparation method I had heard about was Lamaze. It appeared that the only alternative to drugged labor and delivery was the artificiality of patterned breathing and staring fixedly at a focal point. The method did not seem to emphasize the importance of immediate physical contact between mother and child, so I felt that there was a lack of follow-through from the breathing exercises to subsequent treatment of the baby.

I learned about the Bradley method of natural childbirth rather late in my pregnancy, strictly by chance, through an article in the local newspaper. I had, after months of searching, finally found a doctor who was sympathetic to my ideas about how babies should be born and a hospital which would permit me to mother the child as soon as it was born. I was interested in the Bradley course because it seemed primarily concerned with insuring the welfare of the infant by insuring the welfare of the mother.

The Bradley method is deceptively simple. It assumes that normal childbirth is a natural process in the well-nourished mother—and that it is possible even for modern, sophisticated women to follow the lead of other mammals and let the birth process happen instead of speeding it up, denying it, blocking it out, or anesthetizing it.

The Bradley classes were valuable because they clearly explained how today's traditional hospital and obstetrical practices developed—and why these practices are detrimental to the normal mother and baby. I was also greatly reassured by the information about how the baby grows and develops *in utero* and how my body was undergoing changes that were preparing me for labor, birth, and breastfeeding.

Most important to me, however, was that I learned a way of coping with labor that really worked. The progressive relaxation training was something my husband and I practiced together. I would sprawl in bed in the lounging position (my back at a 45-degree angle, arms and legs supported by pillows, each joint bent) while he simulated the pain of a contraction by squeezing sensitive spots at the back of my ankle or just above my knee. I became so expert at releasing *into* the painful stress, trying to go *with* the pressure instead of countering it with muscular tension of my own, that he could exert maximum pressure, sometimes even using both hands, while I maintained my relaxation: mouth slack, eyes closed, breathing calm, body doing no work. I found during labor that this was the only posture I could tolerate, and having to move out of it caused me extreme discomfort.

I felt the first contraction about 3:30 A.M. We reached the hospital at seven and Matthew was born at 11:46 A.M., so I was in labor at the hospital about five hours. I had often wondered, listening to other women discuss their birth experiences, how anyone could endure anything that lasted so long. I discovered, however, that my time sense was strangely altered: I thought I had been in the labor room for less than an hour when I learned it was 10 A.M. and three hours had passed!

I began to wonder when the pain would become really intense, strong enough to make me rely on my willpower not to take any drugs. For, despite the assurances of my husband and other attendants, I was certain I was not doing very well, that I was tense and resistant, and that I'd never make it through transition, the period when the contractions are the most powerful and come very close together. Then I found out I was already in transition!

All the feelings were tolerable. The seemingly endless series of contractions, some of which lasted six minutes as contraction followed contraction with no rest time, never tempted me to take something. I experienced:

- an extraordinary impatience at the sound of anyone's voice, even my husband's;

- some retching;

- not wanting anyone to touch either me or the bed—the jiggling hurt during contractions.

I thought of the women forced to lie flat on their backs, surrounded by strangers asking them questions, prodding and poking them, and I understood why they wanted to be knocked out during labor. Later, I remembered what Bradley had said in his book about animals hiding when they gave birth, and I was struck again by the stores of instinctual wisdom we intentionally ignore.

In what seemed a very short time, I was completely dilated and things began to happen very fast. The contractions changed from tightening to an overwhelming pushing urge. I felt confused at first, but then I realized that in order to satisfy that urge to push I would have to lose my sense of shame about possibly passing some fecal matter and push with all my strength and with my whole body. When I did this I had a sense of elation, a feeling of ecstasy—deep, powerful waves of sensation that I can only describe as glorious and which reached their climax as I pushed the baby out of the birth canal. I was sorry that this second stage of labor was over so soon. How desperately sad that so many women are deprived of an experience that is all pleasure and achievement . . . and, for me, no pain.

The doctor handed me the baby—a whimpering, slippery, marvelous little creature (seven pounds)—who had been born without screams of agony, either his or mine. He was able to nurse while I was still on the delivery table, and then we walked out of the delivery room, Norm and I pushing the little cart they had put Matthew into. It seemed a perfectly simple and appropriate thing to do, although the staff was thunderstruck. I felt stong, alert, and happy beyond all measure."

The Pregnancy-After-30 Workbook details the regimen that proved so helpful to Edie Grossman and the many other women over 30 who have followed it since. Women of any age who follow this program will reduce their chances of obstetrical and pediatric complications to the absolute minimum. My hope is that this book will reassure women about after-30 pregnancy so they can plan their pregnancies free from the fears which continue to condition popular and medical thinking on the subject.

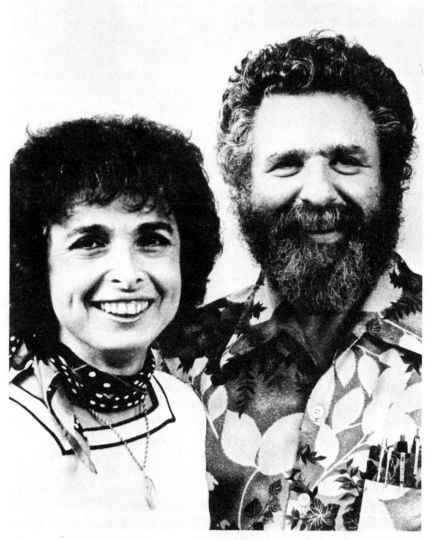

Victor Berman, M.D., an obstetrician-gynecologist, and Salee Berman, R.N., an obstetrical-gynecological nurse practitioner founded the Natural Childbirth Institute NACHIS in 1974 in Culver City, California. Working with other members of a medical team, the Bermans supervise an alternative birth center where nurse-midwives attend the majority of births. NACHIS provides a place where parents receive prenatal care for natural birth, where babies are born, and where the new family receives aftercare.

Dr. Berman graduated from the University of Colorado and the Howard University Medical School. He completed an OB-GYN residency at Margaret Hague Hospital in Newark, New Jersey.

Salee Berman holds degrees from the University of Minnesota, Santa Monica College School of Nursing and is a candidate for a master's degree in public health from Goddard College, Los Angeles.

1
Who Runs a Higher Risk?
A Consultation About
Childbearing After 30

by: Victor Berman, M.D.
and Salee Berman, R.N.

More women today than ever before are considering pregnancy after the age of 30. The latest available statistics show that in the United States, 518,856 babies were born to women over 30 in 1975. Careers other than mothering, later marriages or second marriages, and advances in fertility management are some of the reasons for this new twist in pregnancy statistics.

However, many women fear waiting past 30 to become pregnant. They have been told by doctors and others that they are much more likely to have a difficult pregnancy or a defective child because of their age. Some, when they discover they are pregnant, are advised to terminate the pregnancy for no other reason than their age—even when they have had successful pregnancies previously.

We are often asked if it is dangerous for a woman to defer pregnancy until she is past her twenties. Should every older woman be considered a high risk for developing complications during pregnancy or birth?

First, let's discuss the concept of risk. If you get up in the morning, there is a risk you might not live until evening. If you start to cross the street, there is a risk you might not get to the other side. Some people do not drive on high-speed roads or fly in commercial airplanes because they consider these activities to be unacceptable risks. Others amuse themselves by racing motorcycles and hang-gliding. They feel that the thrill and adventure add enough to the quality of their lives to be well worth the risk. Most of us fall somewhere between these extremes.

Each of us must decide hundreds of times a day what constitutes an acceptable risk. We do this by subconsciously calculating risk-benefit ratios. We evaluate situations and then make judgments. For example:

Is the risk of getting a speeding ticket worth the benefit of getting to work on time?

Is the risk of burning yourself worth the benefit of a warm fire in the fireplace?

Are the risks of having an unhappy marriage worth the benefits of trying for a happy marriage?

The very least of my concerns was my age. When I learned I was pregnant, I felt like shouting the news from every rooftop! Who cared whether I was 23 or 33. I was simply ecstatic. I was healthy and felt great—and that was all that mattered.

When my pregnancy was first confirmed, the doctor who gave me the results just assumed that at 39, I would want to be scheduled for an abortion. I had three older boys already, he said, and, besides, there was a good chance this baby would be defective due to my age.

My husband and I talked it over a lot, and we also talked to my cousin who is a genetic specialist. The cousin was strongly in favor of terminating the pregnancy, and if we wouldn't consider it as a matter of course, he said I should have amniocentesis as soon as possible to make sure there was no genetic defect in the baby. He also said that even if the amniocentesis was okay, there was still a much greater risk of other kinds of problems (like stillbirths and mental retardation) in children born to older mothers, so abortion should still be my first choice!

1

The pleasure of having your first child at the age of 40 is immense. My enthusiasm for getting pregnant was due to a feeling of readiness mentally as well as physically.

I just knew this pregnancy was going to be the best of all. At 33, I was stronger, healthier, happier, and more active than when I was 18, or 23, or 28. I was feeling at my peak, and for this pregnancy I knew how to do everything right.

Perhaps one of my greatest assets was my age. It took a lot of learning through the years to discover just exactly what "doing everything right" was all about. I knew the deck was stacked in my favor this time.

I had my first child at age 31 and my most recent at age 38. Fortunately, I learned how to eat correctly between age 31 and 38. My pregnancy, labor, and baby were all healthier at age 38.

We discovered that our first child had a learning disability. I could not have coped with this development as well had I been younger and less mature in my thinking.

We apply these risk-benefit calculations to everyday, insignificant events as well as to the major decisions of a lifetime. Unfortunately, many of our choices are made with insufficient information in our computers to figure risk-benefit ratios thoroughly. Yet, we take pride in considering ourselves reasoning human beings, and we constantly seek information to help us make better decisions.

When a woman is thinking about having a baby, she weighs risks and benefits, too. In our view, every decision to bear a child is unique. The age of the parents is only one very small factor in deciding whether an individual should consider pregnancy. Many other factors affect the risk-benefit ratio in each woman's case. It is necessary for each individual to know as much as possible about her own situation, physically, emotionally, and socially, before she can decide whether pregnancy would be a high risk for her.

Statistics Emphasize the Risks Older Mothers Face

The published statistics about the problems of women after 30 in pregnancy and childbirth frighten many women into forgoing the experience. While statistics may be an interesting way to look at certain phenomena or to check trends as they develop, usually they do not provide enough information to determine how an individual should be cared for at a given time.

For example, statistics tell us that older women are two-and-a-half times more likely to have an abruption of the placenta (a condition in which the placenta separates from the wall of the uterus before the baby is born). But they do not tell us that all mothers over the age of 30—sick and well, rich and poor, well nourished and malnourished—have been used to set this figure. They don't say that abruptions are the result of poor nutrition during pregnancy, and that many of the older women who experience abruption do so because they have many mouths to feed and, so, eat poorly themselves during later pregnancies.

The point is that an individual woman will *only* become a high risk for an abruption if she is malnourished, but the statistics do not distinguish between the risks of this condition for the well fed and the risks for those whose diets are inadequate. Instead, the statistics present the problem strictly on the basis of age. We prefer to base our expectations for an individual woman's pregnancy on her own medical history and current health status. Statistics alone have little validity as guidelines for the management of individual pregnancies.

The "Best" Age to Have a Baby

We are thoroughly opposed to the concept that age alone should be a deterrent for a woman who wants a child. Many authorities have come up with suggestions for the "best age" to have a baby: 18 to 20, 20 to 25, 25 to 30. Each age group has its proponents, and each proponent can give good reasons for that choice. If a person really had a choice, it might be possible to define one age group as better in terms of a woman's physical health or social development. However, in the vast majority of cases, there is no choice. A woman may be too involved with her personal or professional career to have children when she is younger. She may not yet have met the right person to be the father of her children. She may have encountered difficulties in getting pregnant. Or, she simply may not have been ready to settle down. In any of these cases, there is no choice involved. She waits until she is ready.

This is not to say that waiting past the age of 30 is without obstacles or trade-offs. There are obstacles to be considered in childbirth at this age, but many of these obstacles are slight. Many of them can be predicted, and many can be overcome. Most important, in spite of all the obstacles, the odds are greatly in favor of having a successful pregnancy at almost any age. Support for this point of view comes from our own experience with pregnant women as well as from studies of reproduction in later life. Lawrence R. Wharton, M.D., after studying normal pregnancies in women past the age of 50, concluded that general health is much more important than age alone as a factor in predicting the outcome of a pregnancy. If your health is good, there is no age at which pregnancy should be abandoned due to age alone. Each case must be decided individually according to its own merits.

It is obvious that the longer a person lives, the more likely it is that she will have some kind of health problem. Whether the problem is serious enough to disallow pregnancy altogether, or to require special handling for a successful outcome, is a determination each woman must make after a thorough round of consultations with the medical personnel involved. Specifically, fertility problems of which the couple have been unaware, preexisting medical disease, previous surgery, familial or genetic disease, past pregnancy performance, and any psychological difficulties may present obstacles serious enough to warrant caution in proceeding with pregnancy. A complete medical history is the best tool we have for discovering whether any of these factors are significant for an individual.

Sure, I always wanted to have children and lots of them. But it never occurred to me to have them earlier. I was totally absorbed first with my studies, then with my jobs. In my late teenage years, I had two goals: working with animals (which specifically became racehorses) and flying high above the ordinary crowd to see the world and its colorful people. It took 14 short and beautiful years to satisfy me; then I could turn the page without regret and start a new chapter.

That was when Frank and I decided to have our first child. We both enjoyed my pregnancy tremendously, although it didn't seem to agree with my body during the first four months.

My mother had my brother when she was 42 years old. It was an easy birth, without drugs. My grandmother had her sixth child at the same age. My best friend's mother also had her last child at 42. So I was in no hurry. It never occurred to me to worry about being a high risk simply because I was over 30.

Just when I'm becoming somewhat mature, I suddenly find that I'm also becoming "elderly." Dancers are also considered too old at age 30—burned out bodies due to using faulty technique, doing too much too fast, not respecting the body. Fortunately that's changing, and we are getting more mature dancers—childbearing is changing too. We are becoming more mature. We are learning how to cooperate with our bodies—to respect them.

Dealing with Fertility Problems

Suppose you are an older woman who has been trying to become pregnant and hasn't conceived. What can you do about it? We feel a complete workup with an infertility specialist, not a generalist obstetrician-gynecologist, should begin after six months of trying. It is important for the couple to understand that infertility is a medical problem that they share. To attack the problem most effectively, the cooperation and understanding of both partners, working with an able specialist, is essential.

There is a tendency to regard infertility as a woman's problem when actually there are multiple factors involved, many of which originate with the man. Another pitfall is assuming that any doctor is qualified to handle infertility problems. For many couples, the anxiety and tension that infertility creates require that help be obtained speedily.

The general practitioner who deals with infertility as only a small percentage of routine practice cannot provide the comprehensive services many couples need to determine the cause of their infertility and have it successfully treated. Several organizations now exist to provide information and support to couples with fertility problems. The American Fertility Society and Planned Parenthood-World Population maintain referral services to infertility specialists across the country. Another source of information about infertility clinics is your local medical school where specialists receive their training.

Wait Three Months After Stopping the Pill

Incidentally, we caution women who have been taking birth control pills *not* to try to conceive until three months after they have stopped taking the pills. There have been reports of increased rates of spontaneous abortions (miscarriages) in women who become pregnant immediately after stopping the pill. It may have to do with the changes in hormone levels which the pill induces. We counsel couples to use a diaphragm, condom, or foam during the three months prior to attempting conception. This period allows the mother's body to reestablish its own ovulation cycle, independent of the influence of the pill.

One final point about possible infertility: although there is agreement that fertility decreases with age, various studies show more than half of women are ovulatory up to age 46. Contrary to the popular belief that younger women have the highest fertility rate, these studies conclude that the most fertile group is women between ages 31 and 35. As the accompanying graph shows, only after age 40 does the

Lifetime Reproductive Cycles

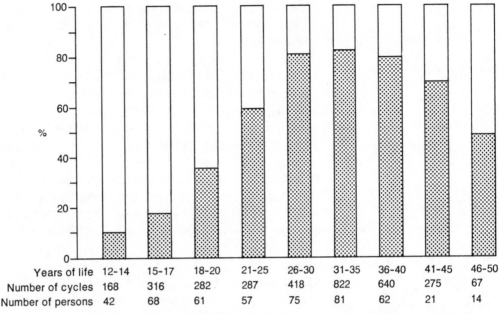

Years of life	12-14	15-17	18-20	21-25	26-30	31-35	36-40	41-45	46-50
Number of cycles	168	316	282	287	418	822	640	275	67
Number of persons	42	68	61	57	75	81	62	21	14

C. E. Adams ARC. Unit of Reproductive Physiology and Biochemistry, Cambridge

Each column includes an age-group of 3 (later 5) consecutive years. The black area represents the proportion of normal cycles.

fertility rate begin to drop significantly. Approximately 50 percent of the women in these studies continued to have menstrual cycles at age 50. Whether or not an individual is still ovulating can be determined by keeping a basal body temperature chart. This procedure can be explained by any obstetrician-gynecologist. Determining whether the woman does indeed ovulate is usually the first step in an infertility workup.

Spontaneous Abortions (Miscarriages)

Some couples are frustrated in their desire to have a child by secondary infertility, that is, losing a baby due to spontaneous abortion (miscarriage) after conception. About one in six pregnancies ends before the baby can survive outside the uterus. Three-fourths of spontaneous abortions occur before the twelfth week of gestation and are caused by defective embryos and/or deficient placentas. Conditions in the mother account for the other 25 percent of spontaneous abortions: fibroid tumors of the uterus (more common in older women), cervical lacerations from other births, abortions, or surgery of the cervix, structural abnormalities of the uterus or cervix, acute infections, and profound anemia. Incompetent cervix, in which the cervix dilates

Rachael was welcome, but unexpected; I was using an IUD at the time. Jim and I had decided to wait before making the decision to have a child, mainly because of our financial situation.

The first realization that I might be pregnant was a combination of disbelief and fear. One of my worries was the fact of the IUD, as I knew there was a chance of a miscarriage. Another worry, the greatest, was the effect my age would have on the child. The statistics on mongolism after age 40 were not encouraging. (Other friends of mine who had given birth after the age of 35 also had this concern.) My third worry was that of getting an understanding doctor. I was new to New York and had to rely on some chance in my choice.

My choice of doctors proved to be the help I needed to calm my fears. Two doctors worked as a team, and although they had different outlooks on some things, their overall approach was professional and gracious, with a willingness to take time to answer questions.

My doctor explained to me the chances of a miscarriage if the IUD were removed or if it remained intact until the birth. I wanted it out immediately. I did have to have a second pregnancy test about a month after the removal of the IUD, because I had no weight gain nor could any movement be detected. This was a worrisome wait, but the test again said positive.

Since I had always been in good health, and since the lab tests continued to prove positive throughout pregnancy, the doctor was encouraging.

very prematurely (often around the fifth or sixth month as the baby begins to grow considerably larger), can usually be treated by suturing the cervix shut until the baby is at term. The suture is then removed and labor usually ensues in a matter of days.

Preventing spontaneous abortions generally involves making sure the mother is in optimal nutritional status before she conceives. Some writers suggest that the father should also follow a sound nutritional program for a few months if a pregnancy is planned. If an abortion is threatening (the mother begins to bleed lightly), *hormone treatments should not be given.* These do not prevent the miscarriage and may endanger the developing baby by causing vaginal cancer and possible sterility in male offspring who have been subjected to the hormones. Resting or maintaining usual activities seems to have little effect on the course of events. If the embryo or placenta is defective, the abortion is a normal occurrence in the order of nature. However, most women find it a disappointing and upsetting experience, even when it occurs very early in pregnancy. Any tissue expelled should be saved and taken for analysis to your physician. If the problem was a defective embryo due to some chromosomal abnormality, the couple may wish to seek genetic counseling before attempting another pregnancy.

A woman who is determined to conceive is likely to ask about the highly publicized drugs being used to improve fertility. If she decides to try them, the woman should be sure that her physician is following every cycle intensively after a very thorough workup. Often, more than one drug is used. One may stimulate the ovaries to release eggs, while another changes the consistency of the vaginal mucus to make it more hospitable to sperm. These drugs affect the basic hormonal balance in a woman's body; they are very powerful and should only be used under the closest supervision as part of an overall plan for treatment of infertility. One well-publicized effect of taking fertility drugs is the increased rate of multiple pregnancies that result.

Twins Represent Exceptional Nutritional Stress

The general impression that a multiple pregnancy automatically presents a higher risk for mother and babies is not an accurate one. Of itself, such a pregnancy does not have to be any more complicated than a single birth. The nutrition of the mother is probably the most important factor in the success of a twin pregnancy. Unfortunately, many physicians have not been trained to view pregnancy as a nutritional stress; so they do not see the twin pregnancy as an exceptional challenge to the mother's daily dietary habits. There are two placentas, or one very large one, to be serviced, two babies to be completely formed, and an elevated metabolism throughout the body. When these needs are met by a diet adequate for twin gestation (we recommend a minimum of 140 to 150 grams of protein and 4,000 calories per day), the mother can expect to carry her babies to term and deliver them at a normal weight (not less than 5½ pounds). When her nutritional needs are met, she does not have to worry about metabolic toxemia, a condition for which mothers of twins are also supposedly high risk.

In our practice, we schedule twin births for the hospital rather than our birth center because of the increased likelihood that the babies will be in unusual positions for birth. This is primarily a problem of "traffic management" since there are two babies and often two placentas for the mother to deliver. We are accustomed to our mothers giving birth to seven- and eight-pound twins, by the way, so the traditional concerns about immaturity in twins seldom confront us. Mother and babies stay the minimum amount of time in the hospital, often just a day or two, and are treated like all other normal cases postpartum.

We strongly advise mothers of twins to breast-feed because of the greatly enlarged uterus and larger placental site which must heal after birth. Nursing causes the uterus to contract rhythmically, clamping blood vessels at the placental site, thus reducing the chances for postpartum hemorrhage. Another benefit for the mother is that her uterus will have returned to its original shape and position in the pelvis by the standard six-week postpartum checkup. Nursing also simplifies the daily baby care routine while providing a built-in time for the mother to rest. This approach to infant care smoothes the postpartum course for mother and babies.

Of course, preexisting medical diseases can complicate pregnancy.

It depends, of course, on the disease we're dealing with. Generally speaking, the severity of the disease and the specific medical management required by the individual woman are the critical factors to be considered when pregnancy is contemplated. The four most common diseases which tend to appear as a person gets older are diabetes, heart disease, kidney disease, and hypertension. They frequently occur in combination. Each can have an adverse effect on the outcome of pregnancy if it is not managed correctly.

A thorough medical history and physical examination

I nursed while my husband was in the hospital for an operation. It meant I had to rush home to do it, but it was a time during the day when I had to relax and I needed that.

before pregnancy is the best course to take. Sometimes, though, women with these diseases become pregnant without planning it; they may not even realize they have a problem. Sometimes it is discovered at the first prenatal visit. In most cases, if the disease is identified early, it can be controlled successfully during pregnancy so that mother and baby do well.

When Should the Pregnancy Be Terminated?

If the disease is severe, it might be reason enough to suggest that pregnancy should not be attempted or, if already started, that it be terminated. This decision can be made only after careful consideration of a given case. It would be based on the opinion of the obstetrician (usually in consultation with one or more other experts, often an internist) that pregnancy would probably aggravate the condition to the extent that it would be debilitating or life-threatening. Not only are these diseases dangerous for the mother, but the drug therapies often required for treating them are also potentially devastating to the unborn baby.

Women who must be on medication for some medical disease or other condition should consult the fifth edition of Goodman and Gilman's classic reference book on drugs, *The Pharmacological Basic of Therapeutics* (New York: Macmillan Publishing Co., 1975), to find out what independent researchers say about the effects of medication on the unborn. The well-known and much-recommended *Physicians' Desk Reference,* on the other hand, consists primarily of articles about various drugs written by the companies which manufacture them—hardly an unbiased source of information! Any doubts you have about the safety of drugs you must take during pregnancy should be discussed thoroughly with the physician. Above all, ask if there are any alternatives to the drugs—and inquire about the consequences of stopping the medication during pregnancy and breastfeeding.

If a prospective mother is on medication for a medical disease, she has to find out if alternative forms of therapy might work as well for her if she decides to undertake pregnancy. One very important factor is the strength of the woman's desire to have a baby. If it is very high, she is more likely to be motivated to follow the necessary regimen to make her pregnancy safe.

Many of the standard tests that comprise part of the monthly prenatal visit are designed to screen for these diseases. Urine and blood tests indicate whether the levels of sugar in the body are normal. Blood pressure checks may indicate kidney disease or hypertension. The heart and lungs should be carefully evaluated. Any abnormalities should be subjected to the process of differential diagnosis; that is, each sign or symptom should be accounted for by carefully ruling out various diseases or conditions which could be causing it.

Hypertension Commonly Mismanaged in Pregnancy

This is especially true in the case of hypertension where many differing conditions can cause elevation of blood pressure. Some of these conditions, like the classic one where the mother reacts to stress, or merely to being examined, with an elevation of blood pressure, are harmless in terms of pregnancy outcome. Others, like pheochromocytoma, a rare tumor of the adrenal glands, can be fatal. Too often, a physician will make a quick judgment about what is responsible for a blood pressure elevation and order an incorrect treatment which can jeopardize the pregnancy.

Recent studies have shown, for instance, that continuing low-salt diets and diuretic therapy for chronic hypertensive women who become pregnant is a mistake. The requirement for the circulation of more blood through the growing placenta demands that the mother's blood volume be permitted to expand during pregnancy. When hypertensive women with no other medical disease are maintained on low-salt diets and diuretics (water pills), this normal expansion of the blood volume is thwarted. Often, a woman's pressure will rise significantly higher as a result of the therapy, and she is much more likely to have a premature baby because the placenta cannot keep up with the baby's growth needs when the blood volume is too low. These diets are also likely to be low in protein and calories, resulting in a mother who becomes malnourished over the course of pregnancy, and, therefore, a high risk for metabolic toxemia and a defective baby.

The essential precept we follow in caring for a mother with an underlying medical disease is that she, too, must meet the nutritional stress of pregnancy. So, any therapy suggested must take into account her special needs for protein, calories, salt and other minerals, vitamins, and a balanced diet. Neither she nor her baby can afford to neglect her urgent nutritional needs, regardless of other medical conditions she may have.

Because I feel like a cornered cat whenever I come anywhere near the medical establishment, I had to find the right kind of assistance. (I even get nervous when an old friend of ours, now a doctor, comes to visit socially.) To add to my problem, I once had an episode of hypertension. Then, when I became pregnant, my doctor informed me I had a benign heart murmur. He hadn't mentioned it in 12 years because he "didn't want to worry" me, but he thought I should know now.

My first visit to a midwife program in a Manhattan hospital sent me on a round of nerve-wracking tests, including X-ray (I was concerned about protecting the baby correctly with the lead apron), cardiogram, and others. The cardiologist said that I should be accepted in the program, but the hospital risked me out.

Then I tried an obstetrician who was a woman. On the second visit, she asked me what I was going to do about my hypertension. I'd better do something, she warned. Hypertension could cut down on the nutrients to the baby, who was her responsibility.

I changed again, this time to nurse-midwives at the same hospital. They encouraged me to check my own blood pressure at home, where it remained within normal limits throughout my pregnancy.

Is Pregnancy Safe After Previous Abdominal or Uterine Surgery?

We are often asked whether previous abdominal or uterine surgery makes pregnancy ill-advised and our usual response is—probably not. The location, size, and strength of the scars from previous incisions must be considered first. In all cases the previous medical record should be carefully reviewed. It is well known that strong scars and good healing do not come about in poorly nourished individuals. If her nutrition has been good up to the time pregnancy begins, the woman has little reason to fear that an old scar would give way as the abdominal wall is pushed forward during pregnancy.

Uterine surgery should not be confused with operations performed on the tubes or ovaries. The latter does not usually result in any increased risk to pregnancy, but surgery on the uterus may weaken the uterine wall to the extent that a Cesarean delivery should be planned. Surgery of the uterus might have been done to remove fibroid tumors, to deliver a previous baby by Cesarean, or to repair perforation of the uterus during a D and C (dilation and curettage) or abortion. In any of these situations, an individual decision must be made. None of them automatically means that a woman must have a Cesarean. The prospective mother should seek other opinions if she is told, without thorough evaluation, that she must have a Cesarean just because she has had previous surgery.

Why Are Cesareans More Frequent in Older Women?

All studies indicate the frequency of Cesareans to be increased in older women. Supposedly the same criteria are used by physicians to determine the necessity for Cesarean in one age group as in another. However, we doubt this is true. Barbara Seaman, in a slightly different context, remarks, "You can't expect objectivity from the sort of people whose textbooks, in this day and age, refer to women having their first child after 30 as elderly primiparas."

Throughout his/her training, there is so much pressure placed upon the obstetrician to think about risks and possible complications during birth that it is difficult to be objective. The physician in practice is further admonished to consider the standard of practice in the community. A medical review board would be most unlikely to question a fellow obstetrician's judgment if he did a Cesarean on a 39-year-old mother, no matter what the reason. However, they might be quick to criticize his decision to "let nature take its

My labor started on a Wednesday morning, and the baby arrived on Saturday morning! I experienced a very erratic labor —stopping and starting. Finally, on Friday night we had to seriously consider going to the hospital within a few hours if labor didn't perk up. The people who were with us felt that due to the size of the baby, the outcome in the hospital could very likely be a Cesarean.

This idea was a shocking fear to me, and almost immediately thereafter, powerful contractions began and continued until the baby was born. I just could not accept the possibility of a hospital birth after preparing so carefully for the nice, warm birth at home. Our baby arrived 5½ hours later. There was very little tearing. It was a WONDERFUL BIRTH!!!

course" were the mother to labor longer than average or to be more than two weeks past her "due date." We think it inevitable that this type of pressure affects medical judgment in the case of pregnant women over 30.

In recent years, Cesarean sections have increased dramatically in mothers diagnosed as having toxemia, which many physicians still view as merely a hypertensive disorder. The problem, as we mentioned above, is that there are many forms of hypertension. Doing Cesareans for hypertension (which occurs more often in older mothers) in the absence of other indications is unnecessary and needlessly dangerous to both mother and baby.

On the other hand, there are a few reasons why the Cesarean rate should be higher in older mothers. Several conditions which result in a Cesarean birth are more common in older women: *placenta previa*, where the placenta lies low in the uterus, is three times more common in older mothers; abnormal position of the baby and *dystocia* (long and painful labor) are also statistically increased. Many women having another child after a previous Cesarean are routinely scheduled for another, rather than being evaluated for this pregnancy. This boosts the rate of Cesareans in older mothers independent of other health factors.

Vaginal Delivery After a Cesarean

The phrase "Once a Cesarean, always a Cesarean," was presented in the *New York Journal of Medicine* in 1916 by Dr. E. B. Cragin. Subsequently, this became a dogma in modern obstetrics. Since then, the validity of this phrase has been challenged numerous times, and today there is a great body of evidence which suggests that, in many cases, vaginal delivery is the better and safer method of management after a previous Cesarean.

The objection to a trial of labor in the mother with a history of previous Cesarean section is the possibility of uterine rupture with its associated increased maternal and fetal mortality rate. There also seems to be an underlying feeling that vaginal delivery simply will not be possible in most cases following Cesarean section.

Let us consider the latter concern first.

In many institutions, women with a history of previous Cesarean section are given a trial of labor. Usually they are selected individuals considered to have a good chance of normal delivery. Figures at these institutions demonstrate that from 21 percent to 91 percent of such women can deliver vaginally.

Let us now consider the subject of uterine rupture.

Most studies report the incidence of uterine rupture in

I was so involved in fighting for a birth with as little medical intervention and as much privacy for my husband and me as possible, that I neglected to prepare for abnormalities or complications. I assumed, from my past healthy medical record and good preparation for the birth, that my first pregnancy and delivery would be normal. In fact, I'd wanted to have my child at home but my husband was against it. He was proven right. After a painful nine-hour labor without medication, I had a Cesarean section and was given general anesthesia. If I'd known I could have had a local anesthesia and been able to see and nurse my child soon after birth rather than waiting a day and a half for the drugs to wear off, I would have tried to have a local. Next time, if the situation occurs again, I'll be prepared.

Vaginal Delivery After a Cesarean

Years	Institutions	Women with Previous Cesareans	Percent Delivered Vaginally
1948–61	Margaret Hague Jersey City, N.J.	2,904	51%
1932–60	New York Lying-In	2,094	21% private 51% clinic
1949-64	13 teaching hospitals in Great Britain	3,429	85–91%

women with a history of previous Cesarean section to be approximately 1 to 2 percent. Most of these cases reflect poor postpartum healing resulting in a weak scar. However, uterine rupture is also much more common in those mothers who have a classical scar (incision vertically through the upper segment of the uterus) than in those with a low transverse scar. Since low-transverse Cesarean section is much more common today than in the past, the incidence of uterine rupture is much lower than in the past.

These are the guidelines we follow in the decision to give women with previous Cesareans a trial of labor:

- Selection of candidates should be individualized.
- Candidates should be seen as early in pregnancy as possible, and regularly thereafter.
- Hospital records regarding type of previous Cesareans, indications for Cesarean, preoperative and postoperative course, and any complications should be reviewed early in pregnancy.
- The physician must take special care to see that the mother is well nourished throughout gestation.

Contraindications to a trial of labor are:

- classical scar,
- two or more previous Cesareans,
- absolute contracted pelvis (fetopelvic disproportion is always a relative phenomenon),
- history of severe infection following a previous Cesarean, a sign of poor maternal diet,
- diabetes,
- fetopelvic disproportion determined by ultrasound or X-ray pelvimetry at term.

A trial of labor should be managed according to these principles:

- Mother is informed of possible risk and is psychologically prepared for the possibility of a repeat Cesarean.
- The mother must be admitted to the hospital as soon as labor begins.
- The mother is prepared for possible emergency Cesarean upon admission (intravenous fluids are started, blood is typed and cross-matched, the operating room is alerted that a possible candidate for Cesarean is in labor).
- The mother is never left alone in labor. The attending physician must be available for emergency surgery at any time.

A few words about fetopelvic disproportion: it is not necessarily a recurrent condition. In many studies, mothers carrying babies smaller than their first frequently had vaginal deliveries, despite previous Cesareans. In several cases with previous section for FPD, women were able to deliver larger babies subsequently by the normal route. This is so in some cases because the position of the baby, not just size, affects the baby's progress through the pelvis.

To summarize, vaginal delivery in mothers with previous Cesareans is not only possible but also a safe and usually successful procedure in carefully selected candidates. There is some risk with this practice which makes extra-careful attention on the part of the obstetrician mandatory; these mothers require intensive care. Physicians encouraging this practice recognize this and, in this connection, usually charge the same fee as they would for Cesarean section. We agree with Donnelly and Franzoni that "Cesarean section is a major operative procedure. If performed unnecessarily in a particular instance, it assumes, and justly deserves, the same onus as that reserved for any type of unnecessary operation."

A friend who was pregnant told me her doctor wasn't going to "take any chances." Since she was over 30 he was going to do a section. I thought she was mistaken—a Cesarean section? That's major surgery and everyone knows recovery from major surgery is more difficult than recovery from a vaginal delivery.

All Women Should Be Familiar With Cesarean Procedure

Most general childbirth education programs offer some information about Cesareans. We feel that every woman should have information about all the options available to her in making the birth of her baby as safe as possible for herself and the child. In some cases, the appropriate choice is Cesarean birth. We require that all individuals using our birth center attend birth preparation classes to prepare for parturition. We prefer the Bradley method because it is the most comprehensive and effective course in reducing the need for Cesareans and intensive care for babies.

It is probably a good idea for women to see a film of a Cesarean birth at some time during pregnancy, just to dispel fear of the unknown. Groups have been organized across the country to promote better understanding of Cesareans and their effects on the mother and family. C/SEC of Boston, the pioneering Cesarean parent support group, can provide literature and guidelines for parents and professionals about the changes they would like to see adopted in the traditional management of Cesareans.

We have been working in our hospital to gain administrative approval for fathers to be present during Cesareans, if it is the mother's wish. So far, we have been successful in three instances where the fathers happened to be physicians. They were important during the births, not because of their medical training, but because they could provide emotional support for their wives that no one else could equal. In cases where the Cesarean is not an emergency and the mother will be awake during the procedure, we like to emphasize the attitude that we are still dealing with the birth of a baby, not just an operation. Having fathers present is one small step in this direction. C/SEC guidelines are fully discussed in chapter 4.

Should You Have Amniocentesis?

Many women past 30 now wonder whether they should have amniocentesis to determine if their baby has any developmental abnormalities. In theory, amniocentesis is a simple procedure. A needle is passed through the mother's abdomen into the uterus. A small amount of the amniotic fluid surrounding the baby is withdrawn. The fluid contains cells sloughed off by the baby. These cells are cultured and analyzed for abnormalities.

In practice, there are potential problems with amniocentesis of which every woman should be aware before she decides to undergo the procedure. First, the mother must realize that not all birth defects can be detected by amniocentesis. Only those abnormalities resulting from genetic miscues can be picked up through this technique. The most common of these malformations is Down's syndrome (mongolism), in which the baby's body cells contain 47 chromosomes instead of the usual 46, resulting in severe mental retardation and often structural heart defects. Approximately 6,000 babies are born each year with Down's syndrome.

While I hadn't planned this pregnancy, I suddenly found myself wanting to keep the baby, even though I was terrified that something disastrous would happen by going through with the pregnancy. So, I decided to have amniocentesis to rule out some of the possible complications and give myself a little peace of mind.

Increasing age has a direct correlation to a rise in the incidence of Down's syndrome. There are two ways of looking at this relationship, as illustrated in the following graphs. Either way, the chances are overwhelmingly in favor of a normal baby. However, if you are one of the 2.5 percent affected, your personal ratio of difficulty is 100 percent.

Incidence of Down's Syndrome in Relation to Maternal Age

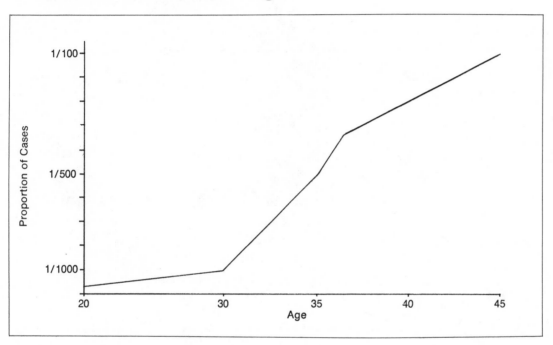

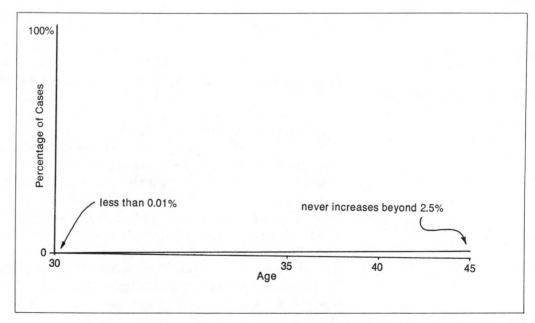

AMNIOCENTESIS

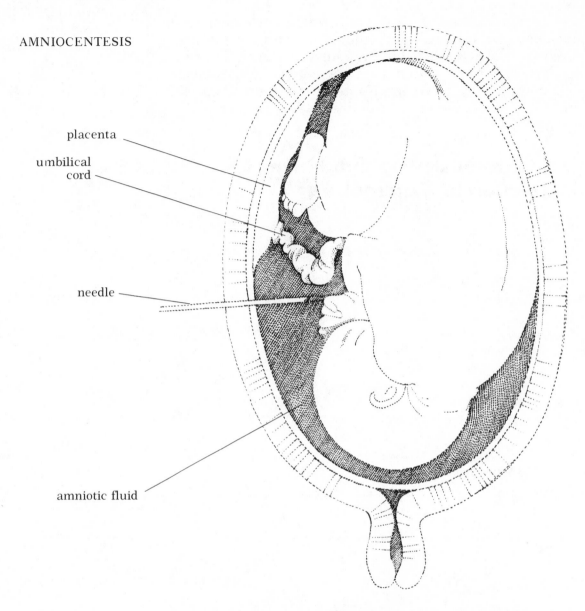

placenta

umbilical
cord

needle

amniotic fluid

The Time Element and Amniocentesis

A second consideration is that amniocentesis can be performed only after the thirteenth week of pregnancy. Before that time there is too little amniotic fluid to make a tap feasible. After the fluid sample has been taken, there is a wait of two to five weeks for the results. This waiting period means that the only alternative, should the baby be defective and the parents not wish to continue the pregnancy, is a saline abortion. In this procedure, a salt solution is injected into the amniotic fluid resulting in the onset of labor. The woman must be prepared emotionally and philosophically for this eventuality since, in our present state of knowledge, there is no way to correct genetic defects. The risks to the woman of a saline abortion in the second trimester of pregnancy are considerably higher than a D and C or suctioning of the uterine contents in the early weeks of pregnancy. If a saline abortion is necessary, it must be done in a hospital with an anticipated stay of one or two nights.

Finally, the mother must realize that the amniocentesis procedure itself is not without risk. The rate of spontaneous abortion (miscarriage) after amniocentesis is approximately 1 percent. Great care must be taken not to inadvertently puncture the placenta, umbilical cord, or baby's body. For these reasons, we do not recommend that amniocentesis be undertaken as an office procedure. Rather, we think it should be done only by people who are specialists and in centers where a setup exists for minimizing the risks involved. Specifically, an ultrasound scan of the abdomen should be done first to locate the placenta and position of the baby. The tap should follow immediately, preferably in the same room, so the mother does not have to walk to another section of the hospital. The National Foundation March of Dimes maintains an international directory of genetic services which lists amniocentesis centers across the country. At these centers, complete genetic counseling is available to parents who need to deal with genetic risks.

To summarize, unless the parents know there is a greater risk for some genetic problem (Tay-Sachs, hemophilia, and sickle-cell anemia are examples) in their families, amniocentesis is not generally recommended until after age 35. In many centers, the procedure is not urged until a woman is 40. In this age range, the dangers inherent in amniocentesis are balanced by the danger of Down's syndrome and other chromosomal abnormalities.

Emotions and Later-Life Pregnancy

Naturally, women who contemplate pregnancy after 30 are concerned about the health of the child they might have, and some also harbor anxieties about themselves. Is a young woman more suited to take care of a baby and grow up with a young child? Does an older woman benefit from greater maturity and better judgment? Are children of younger women more apt to be neglected? Are children of older women more valued and wanted? Obviously, these considerations are individual and differ from person to person.

One mother of three, 33 years old at the birth of her third girl, said, "This child meant more because we thought about the pregnancy more and planned it more carefully."

A 35-year-old woman who had undergone amniocentesis

My husband did quite a bit of research on amniocentesis before the procedure was scheduled. He called the hospital in Manhattan where I had been advised to go for the test and asked how their system was arranged. We found out that the sonar equipment to locate the placenta and position of the baby were in an entirely different building than the office where the actual tap is done! The idea of an hour's delay between the times the sonar scan and the actual tap were done was totally unacceptable to us (we knew it was possible for the baby's position to change), so we had to travel to the only other approved hospital, way out on Long Island, in order to have the amniocentesis.

The amniocentesis procedure was very painful. But, perhaps this was because the doctor had led me to believe that I would feel nothing. Also, they were very blasé about the risks involved—they seemed surprised that we should have any reservations about the procedure. I guess most people just accept the doctor's assurances that the risks are minimal without asking any more questions.

As it turned out, the first tap was unsuccessful, because there wasn't enough amniotic fluid to get a sample; so I had to return in two weeks for a second tap. We went through the entire procedure again, and this time, they were able to get a sample which turned out to be free of any genetic abnormalities. Because I have Rh-negative blood and was never given a Rho-Gam shot after any of my other pregnancies (just one example of the slipshod care given in large hospitals), everyone was telling me I had to come back toward the end of pregnancy to have another amniocentesis to make sure the baby was still okay.

There can be no doubt that I was emotionally more stable and secure with this pregnancy. Having experienced two previous pregnancies, I felt comfortable and knowledgeable this time; I knew what to expect. Certainly, I was calmer and suffered no anxiety or tensions as many mothers do.

As we held our baby girl in our arms (she, by the way, was born without any difficulties), we never were more thrilled in our lives. Our child is the joy of our life. Through her, we experience a total togetherness as husband and wife and as a family.

After our baby was born, all my uncles and aunts came to visit. They admired the baby and paid us tribute. Upon leaving, one of my uncles said, "That's the closest to immortality you can get." I felt the baby had made a great many people happy, and I had never considered this before.

gave birth to a baby who had serious heart trouble necessitating open-heart surgery. She said, "I don't think I could have managed the strain when I was younger. I'm in a much better emotional condition now and am calmer and more able to deal with problems."

We see more younger women separate from their husbands after a baby is born than older women. It seems to us that older women are generally more secure in their parenting role than younger women. These are subjective statements, though. We lack relevant data to support them and would welcome research along these lines.

One aspect of our practice that we feel aids the mother and her partner in coping with the changes pregnancy imposes on their relationship is our team approach to problem solving. Members of our staff include physicians, midwives, nurse-practitioners, family relations counselors, and childbirth educators. We share responsibility for examinations, explanations, and ongoing education during the entire pregnancy and follow-up period. Most important, we encourage parents to take an active part in decisions which affect them and their babies. We try to create a free and open atmosphere so that any kind of problem, physical or emotional, receives attention.

We believe that, for most people, giving birth to a healthy baby will probably be the greatest accomplishment of their lives. So, we like to stress to each set of parents that the responsibility and reward for a successful and healthy pregnancy lies with their efforts. We exist to provide encouragement and assistance in meeting these goals. By the time the baby is due, our center is a familiar place. We have found this approach to prenatal care invaluable in initiating bonding attachments between mother-baby, father-baby, mother-father-baby, and other loved ones and the baby. In this setting, emotional conflicts are reduced to the minimum, and coping skills are reinforced in new parents.

Learn To Cooperate with Your Body

A fundamental attitude we try to convey and support with sound information is this: knowing about your body and knowing how to cooperate with it reduces a mother's risks for problems during pregnancy. The first step in establishing this attitude is getting over the ideas that the birth process is unreliable and the uterus is treacherous. It has been demonstrated to us repeatedly in our practice that by taking good care of the mother during pregnancy, her chance of having a complication during labor or birth is very slight.

In the past four years we have served 700 women, 83 of whom were 30 years of age or older; and 12 of those were over 35. Thirty-four percent of the 700 were having their first babies (primiparas) and 66 percent were having subsequent children (multiparas). There were 8 percent more complications in the 30-or-over group, but more of these mothers were known to be in a higher-risk group in advance. Mothers over 30 who were in our low-risk group had fewer complications than younger mothers. The accuracy of predicting a normal, uncomplicated delivery was better in the older group because they were more likely to have had a child previously.

The percentage of women 30 or over who needed Cesarean sections was the same as in the under-30 group. The percentage who required forceps, induction, or stimulation of labor was less in the older mothers.

The second factor accounting for these outcomes in older clients is that we state our commitment to noninterference in normal labor at the earliest prenatal visit/interview—*and then we stick to it on the day of birth.* In cases where people are not willing to take childbirth education classes or are sure they do not want natural childbirth, we refer them to other obstetrical services. If parents desire more information about our practices and philosophy, we invite them to our monthly open house and encourage them to attend an early-bird class given by one of the area childbirth educators.

At the open house, we invite two or more couples who have had babies with us recently, a La Leche League leader, and a pediatrician or pediatric nurse-practitioner to speak. We present slides and films of some births we have attended, show Dr. Tom Brewer's pregnancy nutrition film, and answer questions informally. We find this gives new clients a better idea of what to expect of our program. It makes them feel more relaxed and encourages those fathers who may feel out of place in an obstetrical office.

We have found that sound nutrition throughout pregnancy, preparation for childbirth, and the avoidance of drugs and smoking are important factors in reducing complications for mother and baby to the absolute minimum.

Drugs During Childbirth

The same need to avoid drugs holds true in actual childbirth. We are convinced that they have no place in *normal* childbirth. This means that in over 90 percent of cases, when the parents have had appropriate care and education, birth proceeds efficiently with attendants having little to do except stay with the mother as she labors. We

The birth itself was a completely natural, undrugged home birth with everything proceeding smoothly. Our new 7½-pound daughter emerged alert with her eyes open and peering into her new world. Immediately after "catching" her, my husband placed her face down on my stomach, whereupon she raised up her head and gazed intently at each of us.

It never occurred to us to go through anything else but natural childbirth. We were very grateful to be able to participate in natural childbirth classes which supported our way of thinking and taught us the different stages and useful techniques during childbirth. We felt confident and relaxed and could hardly wait to see our baby being born.

I couldn't have had better emotional support during labor. I was never left alone; my husband coached me constantly in a very loving way. My two women attendants were also calming and very encouraging. They kept me on top of things and gave me praise as labor progressed.

Without drugs, I felt better after birth, and had more energy than with my previous birth experience nine years earlier when I was drugged.

There is such a difference in an undrugged baby. My son is alert, and was from the start. He nurses vigorously, looks into my eyes with a deep, penetrating stare, and has a calm disposition. He acts like a little person who understands he is loved and cherished. He seems patient and trusting, not fretful.

have a policy of never leaving a mother alone in labor. This sort of emotional support does far more than drugs can accomplish in terms of making labor more pleasant for the mother. In fact, in our experience, drugs introduced during normal childbirth only create problems for everyone involved. They are especially dangerous for the baby since any dose of medication strong enough to have an effect on the mother constitutes an overdose for the baby.

W. A. Bowes and Dr. Yvonne Brackbill in a classic publication, *The Effects of Obstetric Medication on Fetus and Infant* (Chicago: University of Chicago Press, 1970), note that it isn't just the action of the drug itself that can cause problems. These other effects of any individual medication must be considered:

- Metabolites of the drug can augment the effect of a given drug or act differently on the mother than on the baby.
- The drug alters maternal physiology so that respirations and blood pressure may be depressed.
- When the maternal physiology changes, the uterine environment is altered (often there is a reduction in the amount of oxygen circulating to the baby); hence, the baby's ability to handle drugs is reduced.
- There is a natural influence of labor itself on the baby (less oxygen available during contractions, for instance) which may be accentuated by drugs.
- If drugs are given in combinations, all these effects can be sharply aggravated.

When mothers have been attached to a fetal monitor during labor, the effects of drug administration on the baby have been dramatically recorded. This is not a speculative matter. We are interested in doing without drugs because drugs invite complications. For the older mother, recovery after childbirth can be much more difficult if she has to overcome a drug hangover in addition to caring for a baby who has also suffered unnecessary sedation.

Our motto is: Natural Childbirth for a Healthy and Happy Family. After doing everything correctly throughout pregnancy, why stop on the baby's birthday? We believe we are best protecting the unborn child and helping it to realize its maximum potential by not giving the mother unnecessary narcotics, tranquilizers, or anesthesia. In Dr. Brackbill's study contrasting infants born to unmedicated mothers and those mothers who received various types of analgesia, there were significant behavioral differences in the two groups of babies well into the fourth year of life! The American Academy of Pediatrics has stated that there is no known drug which has been proved safe for the unborn child.

Effective Alternatives to Drugs During Childbirth

Proven alternatives to drugs during childbirth include:

- sound nutrition during pregnancy to insure that the mother's body is in the best condition for labor,
- emotional support from caring attendants,
- knowledge of comfort measures and relaxation techniques to remove some of the physical stress of the contractions,
- psychological and physical preparation for the sensations of the birth process, and
- the arrangement of birthing facilities to assist the normal birth process rather than interfere with it (a provision for laboring and giving birth in the same bed, for example).

We are well aware, though, that there are times when medication, anesthesia, and instruments are lifesaving for both mother and baby. In 4 percent of our mothers, for example, a Cesarean section becomes necessary. We explain to all parents that in cases where there is a legitimate need, we have the complete armamentarium of modern medical science at hand. In these circumstances, the risk-benefit ratio of any given intervention must be carefully weighed. The risk of the current complication and its effects on mother and baby must be judged against the potential benefit of some form of therapy.

The problem is that all our drugs and procedures also carry some element of risk to mother and baby. They are not 100 percent safe. This is the time when a mature relationship between parents and medical attendants is a decided plus. If the pregnancy has been characterized by the development of mutual trust and respect, the shared decision-making process is easier.

During a difficult birth, every attempt is made to promote the same qualities of togetherness, bonding, and joy we are used to seeing at unmedicated births. Father is encouraged to cut the cord, and breast-feeding immediately after birth is still the rule. When there has been a complication, it is even more important to emphasize the human values of nurturing mother and baby after the birth is accomplished.

Using the Fetal Monitor in High-Risk Conditions

Many hospitals now try to require all mothers to have their labors monitored electronically. The fetal monitor does nothing to reduce risks in childbearing for women of any age. It is merely a device to detect unusual variations in the baby's response to uterine contractions during labor. It is somewhat analogous to the helicopter flying over snarled traffic with the radio announcer telling that something has gone wrong. It doesn't make the traffic move any better; it just informs you of the situation.

It is interesting that, like so many other interventions in normal birth (episiotomies, forceps, and IVs), the fetal monitor was introduced as an aid in high-risk cases where anything could be expected to happen without warning during labor. Its widespread application to all laboring women has resulted in a skyrocketing incidence of Cesarean sections, since many people who are supposed to interpret the monitors don't really know how to read the machines. Normal variations may be interpreted as danger signs and lead to the performance of unnecessary Cesareans. The monitor also requires that mothers remain very quiet so as not to adversely affect the tracings on the graph paper. This in itself is a detriment to the progress of normal labor since it is far better for the mother to be able to move around as she feels the need.

We follow the recommendations of Dr. Roberto Caldeyro-Barcia, past president of the International Federation of Obstetricians and Gynecologists and a pioneer in research with the fetal monitor. He cites the increased risk of infection to mother and baby when internal monitoring is done. He states that the bag of waters should not be ruptured for the sole purpose of monitoring. In general, we use the monitor only in high-risk situations, for example:

- where labor must be induced due to diabetes, metabolic toxemia, or other medical emergency;
- where labor must be stimulated or augmented with drugs for medical reasons;
- where there is staining of the amniotic fluid with meconium (the tarlike substance present in the baby's bowel at birth) indicating the possibility of fetal distress;
- where narcotics or anesthetics must be used during labor; or
- where labor begins prematurely.

In our practice, where true primary prevention of labor complications is the focus, we seldom need the monitor. Our records for the first two years show the following rates of obstetrical intervention:

Induction	— 2 percent	Anesthesia	—16 percent
Stimulation	— 3 percent	Forceps	— 6 percent
Analgesia	— 3 percent		

The use of the monitor, the need for induction, stimulation, forceps, Cesarean, drugs, or any other interference with the natural process should be discussed carefully with the physician in charge. Only with informed consent can these decisions be made jointly. It is the obligation of the parent-couple to know as much as possible about these procedures so they can discuss them intelligently with their doctor. One reason we strongly favor the Bradley method of childbirth preparation is that these health issues are well aired, so parents feel comfortable making these decisions.

We've said a great deal about the risks of childbirth after 30, but there are a great many benefits to be derived from pregnancy at any age. To quote Carl Sandburg, "A baby is God's opinion that the world should go on." In the old days, it could be said that children were necessary for tilling your fields, caring for your flocks, and providing for your old age. Today, the fields and flocks are cared for by giant agricultural combines, families are being replaced by retirement funds, and the government is caring for the elderly. Who needs children, then? What benefit can be derived from an event that is bound to change the dynamics of a couple or entire family, forcing the reorganization of the daily working life model?

In the Yiddish language there is a word *nachis*. It is one of the most beautiful and expressive words in the language; it means joy and pride in the accomplishment of your children. When a child is born, the way of expressing congratulations is to say, "You should have nachis from your children." When your children are successful, get married, graduate from school, or have children themselves, you are getting nachis from them. The name of our birth center, NAtural CHildbirth InStitute (NACHIS) was suggested by this word. We view this as a very real benefit, a deep enrichment of life.

Another way of describing this benefit would be to talk about the instinct for survival and continuity of the human race, a desire most people have to participate in future generations. What we see in our parents today is a striving for something more than just continuity. They want to have the healthiest children possible and are willing to work toward that goal consciously throughout pregnancy.

We had our first child using the Lamaze technique. The classes were given by the office nurse. We were taught what was going to happen in the course of labor and childbirth.

For our second baby, we had a course in the Bradley method. We learned so much more—and learned we had the right, responsibility, and ability to make decisions concerning our baby's birth.

Is it ever possible for us to appreciate the miracle of life? I gaze at my seven-month-old daughter nursing, and I'm filled with such awe and tenderness and overwhelming love. Does an 18-year-old mother feel this? How can she possibly experience the intensity of life as can an older mother who has lived and seen so much more?

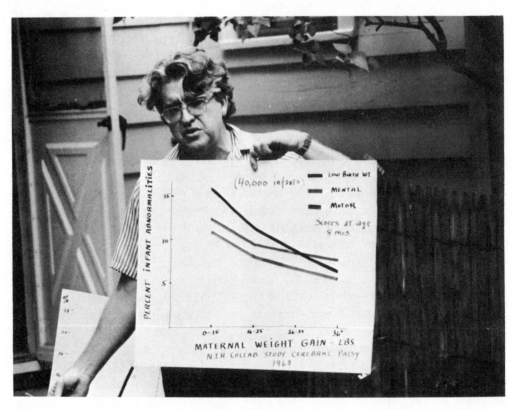

Tom Brewer, M.D., graduated from Tulane University School of Medicine and completed residency programs in general practice and obstetrics/gynecology. A former research fellow at Howard Hughes Medical Institute in Miami, Florida and instructor in the Department of OB/GYN at the University of California Medical School, San Francisco, he conducted a demonstration nutrition education project in the public prenatal clinics of the Contra Costa County, California Medical Services from 1963 to 1976.

Author of Metabolic Toxemia of Late Pregnancy: A Disease of Malnutrition (Springfield, Illinois: Charles C Thomas, 1966), and numerous articles in the medical literature, Dr. Brewer is president of the Society to Protect the Unborn through Nutrition (SPUN), a nonprofit organization committed to the establishment of scientific standards of medical-nutrition management in American obstetrics. He is a well-known lecturer on preventing the nutritional complications of pregnancy.

2
The "No-Risk" Pregnancy Diet by: Tom Brewer, M.D.

No matter how many years you have delayed your pregnancy, no matter how old you are when you become pregnant, there is one proven way to reduce the risk of complications for yourself and your baby to the lowest possible level: Follow an eating program adequate for your pregnancy.

Today, despite a growing understanding of nutrition on the part of many people, the question of what to eat when you're pregnant still provokes debate. And it seems that everyone has an opinion about it—even perfect strangers feel comfortable giving a pregnant woman advice about her diet! Meanwhile, the person most women turn to for accurate information, their doctor, often seems unable to answer questions about nutrition satisfactorily.

Understanding how your body works during pregnancy provides a foundation for an adequate nutritional program. Dynamic changes occur in your body at this time. Some of them, like the growth of your breasts and womb, are hard to miss! But others, because they happen invisibly, are rarely in the forefront of a mother's mind. In fact, few women are ever told that these changes have everything to do with the success of their pregnancies, and that they are of major significance from the point of view of nutrition. Three of these are critically important:

1. the development of the placenta,

2. the expansion of the blood volume, and

3. the increased demand on liver function.

Any pregnancy diet recommendations which overlook these necessary adjustments create problems for both you and your baby.

To separate fact from fiction for yourself, take this short quiz and compare your answers with those provided at the end of the test.

Physically, I was prepared for childbirth. I had always had excellent health, eaten well, and in general, taken good care of my body. After the first pregnancy test, I became an avid reader of anything on childbearing and childbirth. Through reading, I became aware of the tremendous importance of nutrition. I also became aware of the lack of nutritional help from my doctors, and later, from talking with other mothers, from doctors in general. I feel that nutrition should have been the first discussion the doctor had with me, but there was none. I asked him once about foods I should eat, and his sole reply was "Eat a balanced diet." There was never an explanation of food or vitamins.

The nutritional program which I adopted was one of my own, developed from the reading I had done. It was a good program, I believe, and I was quite strict on myself throughout the nine months. I was fortunate in that I had eaten well all my life.

Pregnancy Nutrition Quiz

Section I - Are the following statements True or False?
1. When a woman becomes pregnant, she should cut down on her salt intake.
2. A woman's weight gain in pregnancy must be controlled in order to reduce her chances of a difficult labor.
3. Taking prenatal vitamin and mineral supplements will satisfy a pregnant woman's special nutritional needs.
4. Swelling of ankles, fingers, and face (edema) is a danger sign in pregnancy calling for the elimination of salt from the diet.
5. A baby's length and weight at birth depends on the parents' stature.
6. Brain damage in babies is primarily caused by difficulties at the time of birth.
7. Mothers pregnant with twins should expect them to be born ahead of time and to weigh less than 5½ pounds each.
8. Obstetricians receive training in applied nutrition for pregnancy as part of their residency programs.
9. A high-protein, low-calorie diet is desirable in pregnancy.
10. Pregnancy imposes a nutritional stress only on adolescents and women who were poorly nourished before they became pregnant.

Section II - Choose the best answer.
1. During pregnancy a woman should gain:
   a. at least 24 pounds.
   b. no more than 24 pounds over her ideal weight.
   c. the number of pounds her doctor recommends.
   d. none of the above.

2. Babies have the lowest incidence of brain damage when their mothers gain:
   a. 0 to 15 pounds.
   b. 16 to 25 pounds.
   c. 26 to 35 pounds.
   d. 36 pounds or more.

3. Healthy mothers and healthy babies result when the mother's pregnancy weight gain follows a pattern of:
   a. 4 pounds a month throughout pregnancy.
   b. nothing in the first three months, 4 pounds a month for the next three months, then a pound a week until birth.
   c. ½ pound each week throughout pregnancy.
   d. none of the above.

4. Milk and eggs are good foods for pregnant women because:
   a. they contain all the known nutrients in a balanced form.
   b. they are low in sodium (salt).
   c. they are low in calories.
   d. they are not good foods for pregnant women because they are high in cholesterol.

5. When a woman follows a sound nutrition program for pregnancy, her chances of experiencing hemorrhage and poor postpartum healing are:
   a. increased.
   b. decreased.
   c. not affected in any way.
   d. dependent on her care in the hospital recovery room.

6. The most reliable indicator of a baby's future mental and physical development is:
   a. the Apgar score given at birth.
   b. the physical exam given at one month of age.
   c. the baby's weight at birth.
   d. the mother's weight gain during pregnancy.

7. Nausea or vomiting in early pregnancy is best helped by:
   a. eating plain crackers before arising.
   b. eating high-protein snacks throughout the day and night.
   c. eating as little as possible.
   d. eating foods high in vitamin C.

8. Metabolic toxemia of pregnancy is caused by:
   a. malnutrition.
   b. a poorly functioning placenta.
   c. excess salt intake.
   d. excess weight gain in pregnancy.

9. The best advice for pregnant women about salt intake is:
   a. salt food to taste.
   b. salt food while cooking, but use none at the table.
   c. avoid all foods high in sodium and use none in cooking.
   d. take in no more than two grams a day.

10. A sound diet for pregnancy includes every day at least:
    a. 25 grams of protein and 1,200 calories.
    b. 40 grams of protein and 1,500 calories.
    c. 60 grams of protein and 2,000 calories.
    d. 80 grams of protein and 2,600 calories.

Answers

Section I - *All* statements are False.

Section II -

1 — d	6 — c
2 — d	7 — b
3 — d	8 — a
4 — a	9 — a
5 — b	10 — d

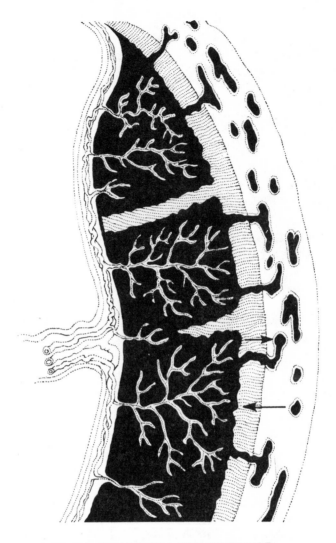

PLACENTA: SHOWING LAKE OF BLOOD

The placenta is an organ unique to pregnancy. It begins forming in the early weeks of pregnancy in order to permit the transfer of nutrients, oxygen, and waste products between mother and baby. The placenta usually implants high on the back wall of the uterus so it presents no barrier to the emergence of the baby during labor. As the baby's need for nutrients increases, the placenta must grow to keep pace. By the end of pregnancy, a normal placenta is the size and shape of a dinner plate and approximately one inch thick, weighing between one and two pounds. It is exclusively a fetal organ, so, after the baby is born and it is no longer necessary, the placenta is expelled along with the membrane sac which enclosed the baby during gestation. For this reason, the placenta is sometimes called the afterbirth.

As the accompanying illustration shows, the placenta allows the circulations of mother and baby to meet intimately but never mingle. The baby's capillaries are continually bathed in a "lake" of the mother's blood. When necessary nutrients are at a higher level in the mother's blood than in the baby's, they diffuse through the one-cell thickness of the baby's capillaries and then procede to the baby's liver for combining into proteins and other building blocks essential to fetal growth. Likewise, when waste products reach a higher level in the baby's circulation, they diffuse back through the capillary network into the maternal circulation and are eventually cleansed from the bloodstream by her liver and excreted by her kidneys. The process of oxygen and carbon dioxide exchange works the same way. Keeping placental function up throughout pregnancy is one of the most important tasks the mother's body must accomplish. If the placenta begins to fail, fewer nutrients are available to the baby over any given period of time, so the growth and development of the baby are retarded.

Added Volume of Blood Is Essential

Sustaining the lake of blood needed to service the ever-enlarging placenta requires a dramatic change in the amount of blood the mother has circulating in her body. At the placental site, it also involves a change in the way the mother's circulation works. Instead of having a closed capillary system, like the baby's, the mother's circulation is open. With each beat of her heart, jets of blood are pushed from her arteries against the surface of the placenta. Blood drains away from the placenta by way of the veins, much the same way that a tub drain catches water when you take a shower. This system is called an a/v (arteriovenous) shunt. Because quantities of blood are free at all times in the a/v shunt, the mother's blood volume must expand by 40 to 60 percent to provide enough for optimal placental perfusion and to keep all her other organs well supplied.

The baby starts to increase in size rapidly at the beginning of the fifth month. As the accompanying chart from Frank Hytten's *The Physiology of Human Pregnancy*, 2nd ed. (Philadelphia: J. B. Lippincott Co., 1971) shows, the rise in maternal blood volume also has a sudden upsurge during that month and continues to rise until just before birth. Any reduction in the amount of blood servicing the placenta impairs its ability to function and, ultimately, imperils the baby.

Nutrition enters the picture when you consider the problem of maintaining such an expanded blood volume. Your body calls into action its own salt-retaining mechanisms (reabsorption of sodium by the kidneys and an increased taste for salt through your taste buds), since salt helps keep water in the circulation.

Rise in Maternal Blood Volume

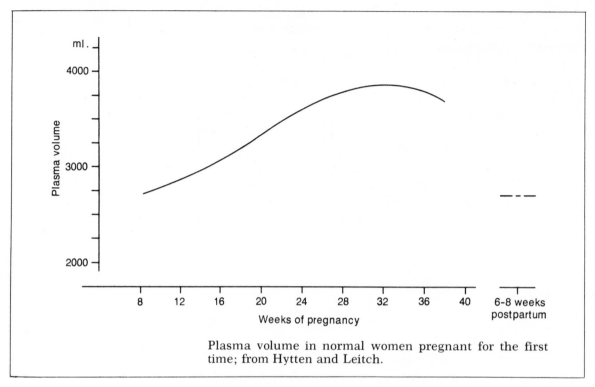

Plasma volume in normal women pregnant for the first time; from Hytten and Leitch.

A second factor is an increase in the synthesis by the liver of albumin, a protein which attracts water into the circulation. A blood volume below the levels needed to meet the demands of pregnancy (a condition called *hypovolemia*) is a serious problem. Not only is placental function threatened, but you also lose your built-in safeguard against dehydration and shock in the event of excess blood loss during labor and birth. Happily, hypovolemia is completely preventable when the mother's diet is adequate for pregnancy, especially with regard to salt and protein intake.

The liver's contribution toward a healthy pregnancy outcome is rarely discussed in childbirth education classes, yet three of its more than 500 metabolic functions have exceptional impact on the well-being of both mother and baby. The first is albumin synthesis. One of the most complicated processes the liver governs, it involves the selective combining of specific amino acids into protein molecules which maintain an appropriate amount of fluid in the bloodstream. Should the liver become damaged, albumin synthesis is one of the first of its functions to be affected. If albumin levels in the bloodstream fall, water which should be in the circulation leaks out into the tissues causing abnormal swelling and puffiness (pathological edema) and leaving the blood volume contracted below the needs of pregnancy (hypovolemia). If the liver malfunction is severe and the blood volume continues to shrink, organs throughout the body are adversely affected by the reduction in blood flow. For instance, in the kidneys, a reduced blood volume results in elevation of blood pressure.

The Liver Must Handle Hormone Overload

A second important area handled by the liver is hormone metabolism. Clearing from the body a staggering load of female hormones manufactured continually by the placenta (the equivalent of 100 birth control pills a day!) requires that the liver attach fat-soluble hormones to other molecules, thus making them water soluble. Then the kidneys can excrete them in the urine. If the liver falls behind in this task of hormone clearance, they can back up in the bloodstream and tissues and reach toxic levels.

Following a pattern similar to that for clearing hormones, the liver must also cleanse the bloodstream of toxins which originate in the lower bowel. Since a slow-down in the process of digestion is a well-known phenomenon in pregnancy, these substances have a more favorable environment in which to develop, thus increasing the stress on the liver.

The only way to meet the stress imposed by this increased metabolic activity is by attending to your diet. The stress on the liver increases as pregnancy advances; so you need more protein, calories, vitamins, salt, and other minerals in the last half of pregnancy than you do in the first half when the baby, placenta, and blood volume are still relatively small. In many ways, the liver works overtime in the second half of pregnancy to meet the physiological demands and adjustments necessary to the health of both you and your developing baby.

Inadequate nutrition, especially lack of high-quality protein, during this critical period can result in severe metabolic derangement and disease. Metabolic toxemia of late pregnancy (MTLP) and abruption of the placenta (separation of the placenta from the uterine wall before the birth of the baby) are two life-threatening complications of pregnancy which result from the hypovolemia and liver dysfunction brought on by malnutrition.

Misunderstanding of the role played by malnutrition in the onset of these and other obstetrical and pediatric problems has blocked efforts to establish standards of nutritional management in pregnancy. Many obstetricians remain ignorant of the advances made in nutritional science

In the beginning of my pregnancy, I thought I should stay thin, so I could get my figure back after the baby was born. I was already eliminating salt from my diet because of an earlier episode of hypertension. After hearing Dr. Tom Brewer explain what is wrong with low weight gain and a low-salt diet, I began eating 100 grams of protein a day plus salt. My pregnancy was comfortable; no morning sickness, and no elevation in blood pressure.

One day we ate in a restaurant near the hospital. A waitress told us of her pregnant daughter's eating habits (she was afraid of gaining weight, subsisting mainly on cheese and ice cream) and of her current bout with pre-eclampsia. The waitress herself had gained 40 pounds during her own pregnancy, and had had no problems with illness during that time.

During my prior two pregnancies, I had been very uncomfortable much of the time and had experienced several problems: severe leg cramps, stretch marks, headaches, susceptibility to colds, intense and painful abdominal muscle spasms, fatigue, and a heavy, draggy feeling. For some reason, my physician had put me on diuretics then, although I never did seem to have a water-retention problem, and I avoided salt. I was miserable: I hurt physically and emotionally, and I felt drained and frequently depressed.

Over the past few years I've "discovered" health and have become very careful of my diet, eating mostly raw foods and avoiding all processed foods or foods containing additives. Throughout this pregnancy, I consistently ate very large quantities of protein—at least 100 grams per day—in the form of eggs, yogurt, powdered milk, brewer's yeast, wheat germ, all kinds of raw nuts and seeds, cheeses, beans, sprouts, and occasionally some fish or poultry. I've always been big on vegetables and fruits, and each day I had at least three servings of fruits and lots of vegetables and hearty vegetable salads. The other foods in my diet varied, such as millet, brown rice, potatoes, whole grain breads, and so forth. In addition, my supplements consisted of a regular prenatal vitamin-mineral tablet, desiccated liver, vitamin C (approximately 1 gram), vitamins A and E, plus extra B_6. My skin glowed; my hair grew so fast it needed cutting every three to four weeks.

over the past 50 years, clinging to outmoded prenatal regimens which do not recognize the nutritional stress pregnancy imposes on every woman. In many instances, these regimens (usually featuring low-calorie, low-salt diets and use of diuretics to combat swelling) were originally advanced as ways of preventing MTLP and abruptions. However, it is now clear that such dietary advice *brings about* the very conditions it was supposed to prevent by inducing malnutrition in pregnant women who may have been perfectly healthy before beginning to follow the physician's advice!

Failure to give every woman correct advice about her diet during pregnancy jeopardizes the mother and her baby by making them subject to higher risks for many of the most-feared pregnancy complications. In additon to MTLP and abruption of the placenta, severe infections, anemia, hemorrhage, and poor postpartum healing are common obstetrical problems when mothers are malnourished.

Lower birth weight and resulting neurological deficits in children are also directly dependent on the quality of the mother's pregnancy diet. Babies who are underweight at birth have a significantly higher incidence of a broad spectrum of developmental problems including mental retardation, epilepsy, cerebral palsy, hyperactivity, and learning disabilities. Babies who die within the first 28 days of life are 30 times more likely to have been underweight at birth.

Maternal nutrition during pregnancy is the single most important factor affecting the baby's birth weight. When your diet is adequate for your pregnancy, the placenta continues to function well up until the day your baby is born, and your chances of giving birth to an underweight baby are almost nil.

Baby's Brain Grows Most Rapidly in Last Two Months

Keeping an adequate supply of nutrients available to the growing baby is critical during the last eight weeks of pregnancy when the baby's brain is growing at its most rapid rate ever. Cells are proliferating and interconnections between them are being laid down. Research done in England over the past 20 years has shown that even mild degrees of maternal undernutrition in these last few weeks of pregnancy can adversely affect this phase of the baby's brain development. So, even the mother who has been eating well up until the last two months of pregnancy can still give birth to a damaged child if she follows an uninformed physician's order not to gain another ounce before delivery.

Focus on Nutrition, Not Pounds

While the number of pounds gained during pregnancy says nothing about the quality of the mother's diet (you can gain weight by eating lots of empty calories or by eating lots of nutritious foods), the National Institutes of Health Collaborative Study of Cerebral Palsy and Other Neurological Disorders found in 1968 that mothers who gained 36 pounds or more in pregnancy had the lowest incidence of low birth weight and brain-damaged children (see chart). For this reason alone, doctors should abandon the practice of restricting a pregnant woman's weight gain to any prescribed number of pounds. Instead, his efforts and concern should be redirected toward insuring that each woman obtains a diet adequate for her pregnancy.

When the focus is on *nutrition, not pounds,* weight gain will take care of itself. Some mothers, overweight at the beginning of pregnancy, may even lose a few pounds during pregnancy when their menu choices are made from higher-quality foods. The idea that every pregnant woman should conform to some ideal weight gain total or pattern disregards the incredible variability of metabolism, activity

Birth Weight Related to Mental Function

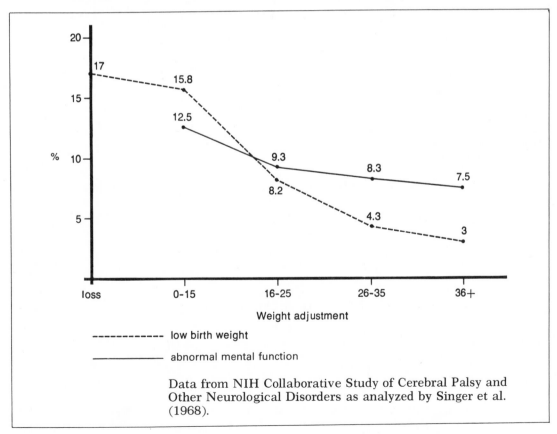

Data from NIH Collaborative Study of Cerebral Palsy and Other Neurological Disorders as analyzed by Singer et al. (1968).

levels, and food choices that can characterize normal pregnancy.

As the accompanying chart shows, British investigators of normal physiological adjustments in pregnancy found that patterns of gain in the last half of pregnancy

Range of Mothers' Weights in Normal Pregnancies and Deliveries

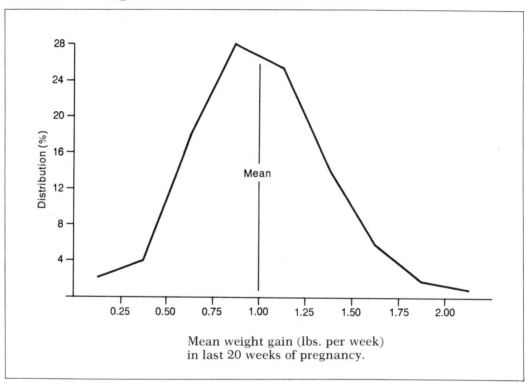

Mean weight gain (lbs. per week)
in last 20 weeks of pregnancy.

ranged from weight losses to more than 40 pounds gained. Since all the mothers included in this study had normal pregnancies and normal babies, it is obvious that pounds gained or lost per se are not the critical issue affecting maternal and infant health. The important factor is what the mother actually eats, day by day.

The foods you eat every day of your pregnancy play a critical role in your health; in the health, growth, and development of your unborn baby; in your labor and delivery; and in the health and future development of your newborn baby. Most medical personnel in the United States today have not been made aware of this fact despite the extensive research done in the last half-century confirming it. Being pregnant, you can't afford this type of skepticism because pregnancy puts a special nutritional stress on every woman regardless of her age, health status, or previous number of children. Failure to meet this increasing daily stress with enough good foods, salt, and water leads to many nutritional complications of pregnancy, including difficulties in labor and delivery, which harm both mother and baby.

Pregnancy Complications Due to Malnutrition

Most doctors and nurses in the United States today don't recognize that a large majority of these complications are directly caused by malnutrition during pregnancy and are hence *preventable!* In fact, the idea of prevention of pregnancy diseases by nutritional means alone is likely to be regarded in all our teaching medical centers as faddism lacking scientific proof. Therefore, all pregnant women who receive prenatal care influenced by this indifference to applied nutrition are at much higher risk than women whose nutrition receives top priority as a routine part of their prenatal care.

If you have passed your thirtieth birthday, you will be considered as even a higher risk from the point of view of several common problems which are directly related to your diet during pregnancy: metabolic toxemia of late preg-

The importance of proper diet cannot be overemphasized. I followed the "No-Risk" Pregnancy Diet, and the difference in my well-being between this and my previous two pregnancies was dramatic. I had boundless energy, no leg cramps, no stretch marks, no varicose veins, no headaches—no problems or discomforts of any kind whatsoever throughout the entire period.

We all know how important good food is to our physical well-being, but I think the emotional factor must also be stressed, particularly during this time of hormonal changes and added concerns. Many pregnant women experience depression and mood fluctuations which are a direct result of poor eating habits. I felt happy, alert, and "all together" throughout my nine months.

Medical research during the last 40 years has clearly shown that the following pregnancy complications can be *directly caused by malnutrition.*

A. For Mothers:
  1. Metabolic toxemia of late pregnancy (MTLP)
  2. Premature separation of the placenta (afterbirth)
  3. Severe infections
  4. Severe anemias
  5. Miscarriages and molar pregnancy
  6. Premature labor and delivery
  7. Prolonged and difficult labor
B. For Babies:
  1. Stillborn babies, especially when MTLP and premature separation of the placenta occur
  2. Lowered birth weight
  3. Prematurity
  4. Severe infections
  5. Hypoglycemia
  6. Birth defects, especially defects of the brain leading to cerebral palsy, epilepsy, mental retardation, hyperactivity, and learning disabilities

nancy (MTLP), hypertension, diabetes mellitus, and obesity. When you understand the role of diet in the *prevention* of MTLP and in the correct management of the other problems, you and your baby will no longer be in this high-risk category. In fact, with correct nutrition and drug practices all through pregnancy, you will be an even lower risk than average.

Metabolic Toxemia of Late Pregnancy (MTLP)

I identified this as a specific disease entity in 1966. It is primarily a disease of the liver and characterized by a history of malnutrition, nausea and vomiting, low blood proteins (especially low serum albumin), and low blood volume (hypovolemia) which causes a marked reduction in blood flow to the placenta, kidneys, and other organs. It

Nutritional Deficiency in Pregnancy

Complications	Control Group (750)	Nutrition Group (750)
Preeclampsia	59	0
Eclampsia	5	0
Prematures (5 lb. or less)	37	0*
Infant Mortality	54.6/1,000	4/1,000

—Adapted from Winslow Tompkins. *Journal of International College of Surgeons* 4:147, 1941. (* Smallest baby weighed 6 lb. 4¼ oz.)

Prevention of Convulsive MTLP (Eclampsia)

	Number of Pregnancies	Cases of Convulsive MTLP (Eclampsia)
Tompkins 1941	750	0
Hamlin 1952	5,000	0
Bradley 1974	13,000	0
Davis 1976	500	0
Brewer 1976	7,000	0
Total	26,250	0

occurs in the last half of pregnancy, more often in the seventh to ninth months, and disappears a few days after delivery.

As a result of the hypovolemia and liver malfunction, the mother's blood pressure rises as the disease progresses, water and salt are retained abnormally, and protein appears in the urine. In the severest cases hemorrhages develop in the mother's liver and brain; convulsions, coma, and maternal and fetal deaths occur. This disease was previously termed toxemia of pregnancy or preeclampsia/clampsia. *Eclampsia*, from the Greek word meaning a flash of light, was used for the severest form of the disease when the mother had convulsions and/or coma. Preeclampsia was used for the nonconvulsive stage characterized by excess water retention (edema), high blood pressure, and protein in the urine. Preeclampsia, as used by doctors and nurses in the United States, is a poorly defined entity, really a *syndrome*, because edema, high blood pressure, and protein in the urine occur commonly in human pregnancy from many other causes than MTLP.

Winslow Tompkins at the Philadelphia Lying-In Hospital reported in 1941 his success in the total prevention of preeclampsia/eclampsia by a sound, commonsense nutrition program for all women who came to his clinics. (See Nutritional Deficiency in Pregnancy.) Reginald Hamlin in Sydney, Australia, was able to prevent eclampsia completely by a nutrition program in the public prenatal clinics of the Women's Hospital, Crown Street, London (*Lancet* 1:64, 1952). Dr. Robert Bradley in private practice of OB/GYN in Denver, Dr. Henry Davis in general practice in Carson City, Nevada, and I in Contra Costa County, California, have had similar experiences. (See Prevention of Convulsive MTLP [Eclampsia].)

True Faddism in Treating MTLP

Failure to recognize the role of malnutrition in causing MTLP leads doctors and nurses down a blind alley of true faddism with the still universal use of low-salt, low-calorie diets; blind weight control to some magic numbers; and the use of harmful salt diuretics (water pills) and amphetamines to suppress the pregnant woman's normally good appetite. This irrational approach to management of the pregnant woman's diet has been termed Thalidomide II because it is so damaging to the unborn baby. I was able to prevent MTLP by throwing out of our county prenatal clinics all aspects of this regimen in favor of commonsense, applied nutrition as described here.

For futher information, contact NATIONAL TOXEMIA

HOTLINE (914) 271-6474. This is a service of the Society for the Protection of the Unborn which provides free consultation about suspected cases of metabolic toxemia for pregnant women, medical personnel, and researchers. Review of medical records and methods of medical management are included in the service.

Hypertension in Pregnancy

Pregnant women whose blood pressures reach 140 systolic and/or 90 diastolic (140/90) are considered by most doctors and nurses to have high blood pressure or hypertension. Since women with MTLP may have convulsions and die with a blood pressure of 140/90 or even lower, such blood pressure readings in pregnancy are always cause for great alarm on the part of doctors and nurses. However, many pregnant women have hypertension without any other sign or sympton of MTLP. This may be caused by essential hypertension present long before pregnancy or it may develop during pregnancy—or be detected for the first time during pregnancy if the woman hasn't had her blood pressure checked for a long time.

A well-nourished pregnant woman may develop hypertension from acute anxiety or psychic stress, that is, from some traumatic event in her life, from being worried about the outcome of her pregnancy, from the discomforts of labor and delivery, or just from having her blood pressure checked by a doctor. In such circumstances the doctor's usual diagnosis is pregnancy-induced hypertension (PIH), which is not a specific disease entity such as MTLP. Adding to the confusion is the current fad of diagnosing the hypertension of metabolic toxemia of late pregnancy and the disease itself merely as PIH.

This is a very important point for every pregnant woman to understand because this current confusion leads to totally irrational and harmful methods of treatment of the hypertension with low-salt, low-calorie diets; blind weight control; and salt diuretics; methods which reduce the mother's blood volume and actually cause a superimposed MTLP. The hypertensive woman must be protected from malnutrition throughout pregnancy like every other woman.

Decreasing the risks to the hypertensive pregnant woman with a battery of complicated and expensive biochemical tests is the modern doctor's preoccupation—without any real concern for the woman's nutritional status. As a consequence, the results of the tests are often misinterpreted. For example, Iyengar in India has shown that the urinary excretion of estrogens in malnourished pregnant women increases dramatically when their nutrition is improved with more good foods. Doctors commonly order such estrogen excretion studies without ever recognizing the role of malnutrition in causing the low excretion of these pregnancy hormones, a result of the reduced blood volume following a low-calorie, low-salt diet and diuretic "therapy"!

No amount of diagnostic testing and/or monitoring of mother and baby in the uterus can insure the adequate nutrition of the hypertensive woman nor protect her and her baby from the disastrous consequences of MTLP, premature separation of the placenta, premature delivery and other nutritional complications—but good foods with adequate salt and water can.

It is important to remember that no matter what medical problems are associated with pregnancy, the nutritional stress remains and must be met every day. Low-calorie, low-salt diets; weight control; and salt diuretics are generally *contraindicated* in hypertensive women with a rare exception: when the woman's blood volume is abnormally increased as in severe kidney diseases or congestive heart failure. Such women must be treated in the hospital.

Other rare medical causes of hypertension such as malignant hypertension, brain tumors, and *pheochromocytoma* (a rare tumor of the adrenal gland) also require careful medical attention in a hospital. Except for these rare medical diseases, a woman hospitalized for hypertension, with or without MTLP, must refuse the low-calorie, low-salt diet and diuretic regimen which will directly harm her and her unborn baby.

Diabetes Mellitus in Pregnancy

That good nutrition is the key to successful outcome of pregnancy is nowhere better demonstrated than in women with diabetes mellitus. In Philadelphia, Garfield Duncan, M.D., for years a leading expert in diabetes, was able to prevent metabolic toxemia of late pregnancy (MTLP) in diabetic pregnant women by good management. He advocated each woman have 2 grams of high-quality protein per kilogram of body weight (about 120 grams for the average woman) and at least 2,200 calories daily. Insulin requirements vary greatly; each woman needs the care of an internist to help the obstetrician in diabetic management which must be individualized. Adequate exercise is of great value in controlling diabetes during pregnancy.

We know that poorly controlled, malnourished diabetic women often develop MTLP, fatty liver, stillborn babies, congenital anomalies, excess fluid in the amniotic sac (hydramnios), severe infections in both mother and baby, and acidosis with excess ketone bodies in blood and urine.

It is also clear that low-salt diets, low-calorie diets, and salt diuretics are harmful to the pregnant diabetic and can quickly lead to dehydration, lowered blood volume (hypovolemia), and even to a superimposed MTLP. Diuretics can cause direct damage to the pancreas and must be avoided by all pregnant diabetics. There is no scientific evidence that female hormones (progesterone and estrogens) are of any value in the management of diabetic pregnancies; their harmful effects are being widely recognized today. (See Barbara and Gideon Seaman's *Women and the Crisis in Sex Hormones*, New York: Rawson, 1977.)

Obesity in Pregnancy

The key to understanding the risk of obesity in pregnancy is the concept of the adequate no-risk diet. If you are overweight when you become pregnant, there is no real increased risk *if you can eat an adequate diet all through pregnancy*. This idea flies in the face of convention in the United States, where the obese woman is arbitrarily branded a high risk for developing metabolic toxemia of late pregnancy (MTLP) and for having a hard time in labor and delivery. Such a woman who is harassed by doctors and nurses into starving herself and her unborn baby via the low-calorie, low-salt diet and diuretic regimen *does then, in fact, become a high risk as predicted*. Her pregnancy is made miserable by constant reminders about the supposed hazards of being overweight while she is told nothing about the real hazards of malnutrition for herself and for her baby.

Obese women are, in fact, protected in a sense from one important kind of malnutrition during pregnancy: calorie deficiency. It has been shown in thin, underweight women with few fat stores to draw on that there is an increased risk of MTLP, low birth weight, and brain damage in their babies. If the obese woman eats a good diet, with adequate proteins, carbohydrates, vitamins, salt, and other minerals, she may actually lose a few pounds during pregnancy while producing a healthy, full-term baby and remain in good health herself. This is not achieved by worrying over pounds gained but rather by focusing on the quality and adequacy of her diet.

Weight Gain, Dietary Salt, and Water Retention (Edema) in Pregnancy

How much weight should a woman gain during a normal pregnancy? This is a common question which has

About the sixth month of my pregnancy, the doctor said I had gained too much weight and it was important I cut down. He gave me a diet printed by a drug company. Fortunately, I can't follow diets. Every time I went for a prenatal appointment, he would feel my legs for swelling and look very concerned.

worried women in the United States for a long time. It is clear now that normal pregnancy can happen over a wide range of weight gain. As we have seen, obese women may lose a few pounds while following an adequate, balanced diet, while thin, underweight women may normally gain 50 or more pounds. Women with twins who have full-term pregnancies often gain over 60 pounds with normal pregnancy outcomes for both mother and babies.

We know that pounds of weight gain are of minor importance compared to the adequacy of the diet for the individual pregnant woman. There is no scientific basis for the universal fad of setting up any magic numbers or patterns of weight gain as goals in human pregnancy nutrition. If such a weight limit in numbers is set up arbitrarily, the danger comes when the pregnant woman reaches or exceeds the numbers too early. She thus may be coaxed or threatened into starving herself and her unborn baby during the last critical months and weeks when the nutritional stress is greatest in terms of quantity.

In my clinics through some 7,000 pregnancies, among women never given any numbers of pounds as goals, who were constantly encouraged to eat good foods in response to appetite and to salt their food to taste, where salt restriction and salt diuretics were not used, the usual weight gains in normal pregnancies fell in the 35- to 45-pound range. Normal pregnancies were observed in women who lost five pounds and in women who gained 80 pounds. About 50 percent of normal women gain 20 pounds by the end of the fifth month.

Margaret Robinson, an OB/GYN doctor in London at St. Thomas Hospital, showed us how important dietary salt is for human pregnancy to maintain the health of mother, baby, and placenta. (See the graph Salt in Pregnancy.) She found that salt tablets would usually relieve leg cramps in pregnancy and that depriving women of salt led to an infant death rate twice as high as that observed in women encouraged to eat salt during the entire pregnancy.

With a thousand women in each group, "low salt" and "high salt," the findings were highly significant, if sad. Among women in the low-salt group, there was 2½ times more toxemia of pregnancy and two times more premature separation of the placenta. Twice as many babies died in the low-salt diet group, among women told experimentally to restrict their intakes of salt and salty foods. It is incredible that 20 years after this study, low-salt diets remain in virtually universal use by physicians giving prenatal care.

Normal pregnant women, especially in the last half of pregnancy, retain water to such an extent that they experi-

At 5 feet, 8 inches, I gained 50 pounds, from 125 to 175, and felt great except for severe nausea in early pregnancy; the gain was all on good food, of course. The baby weighed 9 pounds, 15 ounces and I lost 20 pounds total at birth. He is four months old now, and I have continued to eat well for breastfeeding and have still lost 5 pounds. The rest will gradually come off as I continue nursing.

With this pregnancy I ate my foods salted, and I loved it. I never had any unusual swelling anywhere on my body. During the very hot days of early summer, after I had been standing and working most of the day, my ankles would swell slightly, but by the next morning, they'd be back to normal. All told, I gained about 35 pounds—but it was a solid, comfortable 35 pounds. Everyone said I looked wonderful, and I felt marvelous in every respect.

I had no leg cramps with this pregnancy due to my adequate salt consumption and no diuretics.

Salt in Pregnancy

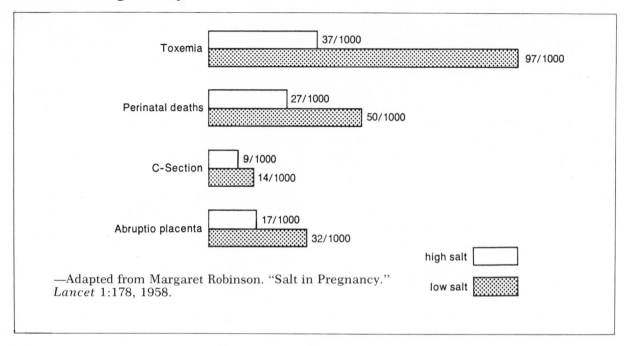

Toxemia   37/1000   97/1000

Perinatal deaths   27/1000   50/1000

C-Section   9/1000   14/1000

Abruptio placenta   17/1000   32/1000

high salt

low salt

—Adapted from Margaret Robinson. "Salt in Pregnancy." *Lancet* 1:178, 1958.

I had less swelling this pregnancy using salt than with my first pregnancy when I restricted salt and used diuretics.

ence swelling of their feet and ankles, fingers and hands, and even of the face. This normal water retention, caused by physiologic changes in the body (see chapter 4), is often mistaken for water retention associated with malnutrition and MTLP. This leads to a great deal of confusion among pregnant women, doctors, and nurses alike. Deficiencies of protein, calories, certain vitamins, salt, and water can all lead to abnormal water retention—not just excess salt in the diet!

Dietary salt restriction is therefore completely irrational in both toxemic edema and normal, physiologic edema. In MTLP, scientific treatment involves correcting the dietary deficiencies with good foods and salt when indicated while physiological edema requires no treatment. The use of low-salt diets coupled with salt diuretics represents a grave error which has not been recognized and corrected by the medical profession. Therefore, each pregnant woman must take responsibility for her own good nutrition. This is easy to accomplish with a proper understanding of these controversial questions of weight gain, water retention, and dietary salt.

The "no-risk" pregnancy diet provides all the nutrients you need by eating to appetite from the four basic food groups and resisting the temptation to substitute less-nutritious foods. By seeing that you eat well, you protect yourself and your baby from the known hazards of malnutrition during pregnancy.

The "No-Risk" Pregnancy Diet*

When you are pregnant, you need more of good-quality foods than when you are not pregnant. To meet your own needs and those of your developing baby, you must have, *every day*, at least:

1. One quart (four glasses) of milk—any kind: whole milk, low-fat, skim, powdered skim, or buttermilk. If you do not like milk, you can substitute one cup of yogurt for each cup of milk

2. Two eggs

3. Two servings of fish, shellfish, chicken or turkey, lean beef, veal, lamb, pork, liver, or kidney

   Alternative combinations include:
   Rice with: beans, cheese, sesame seeds, milk
   Cornmeal with: beans, cheese, tofu, milk
   Beans with: rice, bulgur, cornmeal, wheat noodles, sesame seeds, milk
   Peanuts with: sunflower seeds, milk
   Whole wheat bread or noodles with: beans, cheese, peanut butter, tofu, milk

   For each serving of meat, you can substitute these quantities of cheese:

Brick	—4 oz.	Longhorn	—3 oz.
Camembert	—6 oz.	Muenster	—4 oz.
Cheddar	—3 oz.	Monterey Jack	—4 oz.
Cottage	—6 oz.	Swiss	—3 oz.

4. Two servings of fresh, green leafy vegetables: mustard, beet, collard, dandelion or turnip greens, spinach, lettuce, cabbage, broccoli, kale, Swiss chard

5. Five servings of whole-grain breads, rolls, cereals, or pancakes: Wheatena, bran flakes, granola, shredded wheat, wheat germ, oatmeal, buckwheat or whole wheat pancakes, corn bread, corn tortillas, corn or bran or whole wheat muffins, waffles, brown rice

6. Two choices from: a whole potato (any style), large green pepper, orange, grapefruit, lemon, lime, papaya, tomato (one piece of fruit or one large glass of juice)

7. Three pats of margarine, vitamin A-enriched, or butter, or oil

Also include in your diet:

8. A yellow- or orange-colored vegetable or fruit five times a week

9. Liver once a week, if you like it

10. Table salt: SALT YOUR FOOD TO TASTE

11. Water: drink to thirst

*It is not healthy for you and your unborn baby to go
even 24 hours without good food!*

Note: Vitamin supplements are in routine use in prenatal care; they do not take the place of a sound, balanced diet of nutritious foods.

---

*For a reprint, send 25¢ and a stamped, self-addressed envelope to: Society for Protection of the Unborn through Nutrition (SPUN), Suite 603, 17 North Wabash, Chicago, IL 60602. Bulk rates upon request.

References

Antonov, A. N. "Children born during the siege of Leningrad." *J. Pediatrics* 30:250, 1947.

Bletka, M. et al. "Volume of whole blood and absolute amount of serum proteins in the early stages of late toxemias of pregnancy." *Amer. J. Obstet. Gynecol.* 106:10, 1970.

Brewer, T. H. "Limitations of diuretic therapy in the management of severe toxemia: significance of hypoalbuminemia." *Amer. J. Ob. Gyn.* 83:1352, 1962.

Brewer, T. H. *Metabolic Toxemia of Late Pregnancy: A Disease of Malnutrition.* Springfield: Thomas, 1966.

Brewer, T. H. "Metabolic toxemia of late pregnancy: a disease entity." *Gynaecologia* 167:1, 1969.

Brewer, T. H. "Human pregnancy nutrition: an examination of traditional assumptions." *Aust. N.Z.J. Obstet. Gynaecol.* 10:87, 1970.

Brewer, T. H. "Human maternal-fetal nutrition." *Obstet. Gynecol.* 40:868, 1972.

Brewer, T. H. "Consequences of malnutrition in human pregnancy." *Ciba Review: Perinatal Medicine,* 1975, pp. 5, 6. (Ciba-Geigy, Basel)

Brewer, Tom. "Toxemia—a disease of prejudice?" *World Med. J.* 21:70, 1974.

Brewer, Tom. "Iatrogenic starvation in human pregnancy." *Medikon* 4:14, 1974. (Ghent)

Brewer, Tom. "Role of malnutrition in pre-eclampsia and eclampsia." (Editor's title to a letter) *Amer. J. Obstet. Gynecol.* 125:281, 1976.

Burke, Bertha et al. "Nutrition studies during pregnancy." *Amer. J. Obstet. Gynecol.* 46:38, 1943.

Chesley, Leon. "Plasma volume and red cell volume in pregnancy." *Amer. J. Obstet. Gynecol.* 112:440, 1972.

Cloeren, Stella et al. "Hypovolemia in toxemia of pregnancy: plasma expander therapy." *Arch Gynak.* 215:123, 1973.

Dobbing, John. "The later growth of the brain and its vulnerability." *Pediatrics* 53:2, 1974.

Eastman, N. J., & Jackson, E. "Weight relationships in pregnancy." *Ob. Gyn. Survey* 23:1003, 1968.

Ebbs, John H. et al, "The influence of improved nutrition upon the infant." *Canadian Med. Assoc. J.* 46:6, 1942.

Ferguson, J. H. "Maternal death in the rural South." *J.A.M.A.* 146:1388, 1950.

Hamlin, R. H. J. "The prevention of eclampsia and pre-eclampsia." *Lancet* 1:64, 1952.

Higgins, Agnes C. "Nutritional status and the outcome of pregnancy." *J. Canadian Dietet. Assoc.* 37:17, 1976.

Hytten, Frank. *The Physiology of Human Pregnancy.* 2nd ed. Philadelphia: J. B. Lippincott, 1971.

Mellanby, Edward. "Nutrition and childbearing." *Lancet* 2:1131, 1933.

Pike, Ruth. "Sodium intake during pregnancy." *J. Amer. Dietet. Assoc.* 44:176, 1964.

Platt, B. S., & Stewart, R. J. "Reversible and irreversible effects of protein-calorie deficiency on the central nervous system of animals and man." *World Rev. Nutri. Dietet.* 13:43, 1971.

Robinson, Margaret. "Salt in pregnancy." *Lancet* 1:178, 1958.

Ross, R. A. "Relation of vitamin deficiency to toxemias of pregnancy." *South. Med. J.* 28:120, 1935.

Seaman, Barbara & Gideon. *Women and the Crisis in Sex Hormones.* New York: Rawson, 1977.

Strauss, M. B. "Observations on etiology of toxemias of pregnancy." *Am. J. Med. Sci.* 190:811, 1935.

Williams, Sue R. *Nutrition and Diet Therapy.* 2nd ed. St. Louis: Mosby, 1973.

Recommended Reading

1. Brewer, Gail Sforza. *What Every Pregnant Woman Should Know: The Truth about Diets and Drugs in Pregnancy.* New York: Random House, 1977.
2. Brewer, Tom, and Hodin, Jay. "Why Women Must Meet the Nutritional Stress of Pregnancy." *Twenty-First Century Obstetrics Now* Vol. 2, 1977.
3. Cannon, Walter B. *The Wisdom of the Body.* Reissue of 1939 ed. New York: W. W. Norton, 1963.

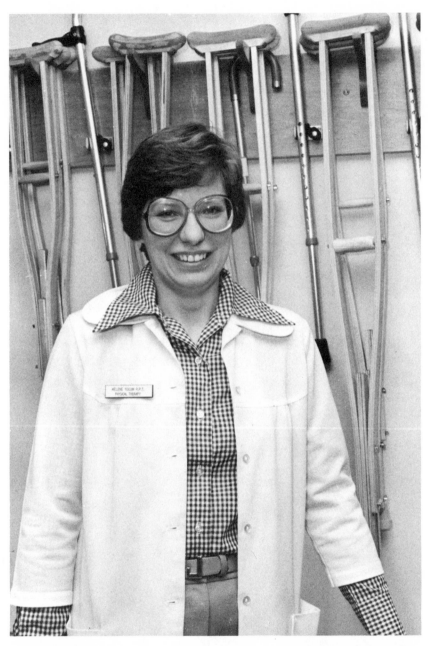

Helene Yocum is vice-chairman for The Section on Obstetrics/ Gynecology of the American Physical Therapy Association. As a childbirth educator trained in the Bradley method, Ms. Yocum gives private prenatal classes. She also teaches postpartum exercise classes at the Geisinger Medical Center in north central Pennsylvania. Helene Yocum, who is married to physical therapist and photographer Vince Basile, resides in Orangeville, Pennsylvania.

3

Movement for a New Life   by: Helene Yocum, R.P.T.

The pregnant woman of any age moves to the rhythms of the new life within her. Clearly, she is experiencing the most amazing physiological changes that the healthy human body can undergo. Many of these changes affect facts about her physical self she has long since come to take for granted: weight, posture, balance, flexibility, muscle tone, and energy level, for example. It is important from the psychological and the physical points of view that she take pleasure and pride in her emerging maternity. A program of basic exercise can contribute much to both kinds of well-being.

Exercise as a way to improve the body's physiological parameters in pregnancy has been recognized since the ancient Greeks. One can read of their special prenatal gymnastics which were taught to all Greek schoolgirls in preparation for their future pregnancies. Today's exercise prescriptions are based on years of research on muscle chemistry, heart and lung physiology, and the effects of the central nervous system on muscle groups. When these are combined with the principles of physics, mechanics, and bioengineering, it might seem that exercise has become an exact science. Most clinical investigations of exercise are carried out using healthy male athletes, a small number use women who are not pregnant, and virtually none involve the pregnant woman. So, common sense and appreciation of the unique body dynamics of pregnancy are our best guides in devising a group of exercises for this period in a woman's life. The goal throughout pregnancy is to maximize physical comfort and prepare the muscles you will use in giving birth. Postpartum, you, like all women, should have a specific program to restore muscle and joint alignment, plus some suggestions about incorporating exercise into daily life so you stay fit even when you're not pregnant.

I was running six laps on a quarter-mile track before I got pregnant, and after that I ran some until my seventh month. I even lumbered around the track in my ninth month, to prove I could do it. I think I should have run more. What better way to prepare for the average woman's greatest challenge than by running?

Comfort Measures

There is a litany of nagging physical discomforts pregnant women are traditionally prone to incur: backache, fatigue, indigestion, swelling, leg cramps, hemorrhoids, and others. Older women may have these conditions before they become pregnant, as the result of years spent sitting at desks in offices or standing for long periods of time at other types of work. Women who have already borne children may suffer some of them because they were not adequately

I really hate exercise, but during pregnancy I made myself do the pelvic rocking and squatting. I have no varicose veins after three pregnancies!

educated about how to take care of their bodies during and after pregnancy. Even women who are physically fit at the beginning of pregnancy can develop these problems if they do not take into account two important changes in their bodies.

First, throughout pregnancy, the body responds to two hormones, prolactin and relaxin, which loosen and soften the ligaments and connective tissue surrounding muscle fibers. One of the first signs that these hormones are at work is the slightly bulging tummy many women notice long before the uterus itself has enlarged enough to push the abdominal wall outward. This early pregnancy expansion results from the slackening of the abdominal muscles themselves. Similar relaxation takes place at every joint. To avoid undue strain on these softened junction points, and perhaps prevent a lifetime of back trouble, it is important to refrain from standard calisthenics designed for the non-pregnant. Instead, emphasis should be placed on bodywork which takes advantage of the mother's newfound flexibility, a factor she will find very important in actually giving birth.

The second change which predisposes one to physical discomfort is the increasing size and weight of the uterus and its contents. Relaxation of the abdominal muscles, coupled with softening of the ligaments of the vertebral column of the spine, allows the heavy uterus to pull the spine into an exaggerated curve. The muscles at the lower end of the back become tense from doing the majority of the work in supporting the added weight, causing the most common discomfort, backache. Other problems result when this posture is not corrected. Irritation of the sciatic nerve (the one which travels through the buttocks down to the back of the knee), neck tension from slumped shoulders, shallow breathing from compressed lungs, and leg and foot exhaustion from improper weight distribution are classic examples of posture-related problems. Correction of posture faults, which may also be present before pregnancy, is essential for maximum comfort during pregnancy.

Learn the Pelvic Tilt

Since there is a tendency for the pelvis to tip forward as the uterus enlarges, the simplest way to combat pregnancy backache is to keep the pelvis tilted backward. When this is done, the abdominal muscles must contract and the lower back muscles must stretch. So, excessive stretching of the stomach and excessive tensing of the lower back are eliminated. In addition, the spinal column is realigned along its entire length.

Pelvic Tilt

Slumped Posture: Upright Posture:

HEAD

If neck sags,   Straighten neck and
chin pokes forward and   tuck chin in so
whole body slumps.   body lines up.

SHOULDERS AND CHEST

Slouching cramps   Lift up through the
the rib cage and   rib cage and
makes breathing   pull back the
difficult, possibly   shoulder girdle.
causing indigestion.   Roll arms out.

ABDOMEN, BUTTOCKS, AND UTERUS

Slack muscles   Contract abdominals
= hollow back.   to flatten back.
Pelvis tilts   Tuck buttocks under
forward, causing   and tilt pelvis back.
backache and strained
abdominal muscles.

KNEES

If pressed back, you   Bend to ease body
strain joints, and   weight over feet.
push your pelvis
forward.

FEET

Weight on inner   Distribute body
borders strains   weight through
arches and calves,   center of
causing leg aches.   each foot.

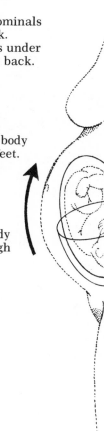

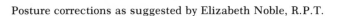

Posture corrections as suggested by Elizabeth Noble, R.P.T.

PELVIC TILT SERIES

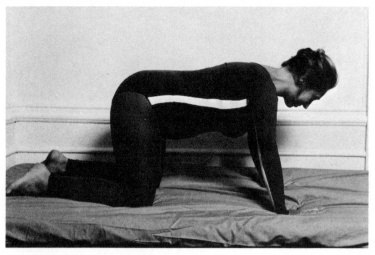

Neutral: back straight

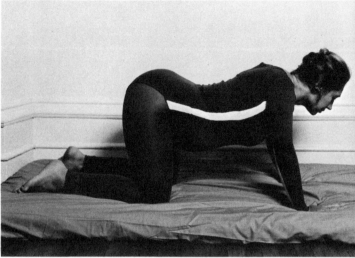

Released: uterus sagging

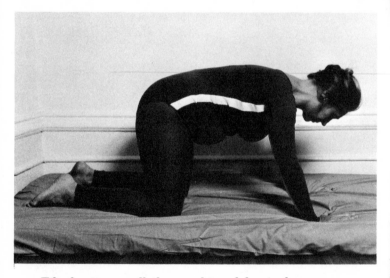

Tilted: uterus pulled up and in; abdominals
and buttocks tightened

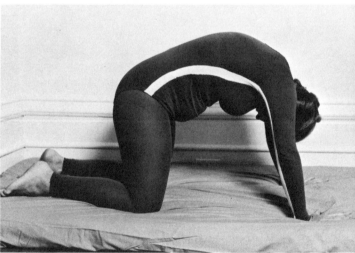

Humped: shoulders being used, not pelvis

The Pelvic Tilt, an exercise which can be done on your
back, on all fours, while sitting or standing, is one of the
best ways to prevent backache or alleviate it if it is already
bothering you. Learning the Pelvic Tilt is easiest for most
women if they lie flat on their backs, with arms resting at
sides, knees bent, and feet flat on the floor. It is helpful to
have a partner to work with the first few times. You will
notice a small space between the floor and your lower back
when you first assume the Pelvic Tilt position. Have your

partner place his/her hand flat on the floor in that space, then push your lower back flat against the hand. You will notice that the adjustment is a very small one, very specifically localized in the lower back. Now allow your back to assume its beginning position, have your partner remove his/her hand and repeat the above so your spine is flat on the floor. Hold for a count of five.

When you have the basic movement very clearly in mind, you can add tummy and buttocks to the exercise:

1. tighten abdomen and hold;
2. tighten buttocks and hold;
3. tilt pelvis so spine is flat;
4. hold a full five seconds, while exhaling
    and counting out loud to five;
5. release just abdominals;
6. release just buttocks; and
7. release pelvis.

Repeat five times, at least twice a day. The Pelvic Tilt is also a gentle exercise for postpartum restitution of tone to the abdomen and buttocks, as well as for treatment of the backache many new mothers experience from carrying their babies around in their arms for prolonged periods of time.

At work, every chance I got I would get down on my hands and knees and do the Pelvic Tilt. If anyone came into the office at these times, I would appear to be looking for my pen which I pretended I had just dropped.

Some women prefer to do the Pelvic Tilt on all fours, especially toward the end of pregnancy when lying on the back can be uncomfortable. This position for doing the Pelvic Tilt has been taught incorrectly in many childbirth education classes, with mothers humping up their backs then doing an exaggerated release (called "the cat and the cradle"). Remember that the movement is really quite small, the objective being to stretch only the overworked lower back muscles.

The Pelvic Tilt can also be done while sitting or standing. Sit on the edge of a chair and rock back and forth until you feel relief. When standing, place your feet about ten inches apart, lean forward slightly with hands resting on something at counter height, then tilt pelvis as described above. The Pelvic Tilt can be done as long as you like, as many times a day as you need for your own comfort. It is very relaxing to do it before sleep, after a leisurely warm bath.

The vast majority of back discomforts can be alleviated by application of heat (tub bath, shower massage, hot water bottle, heating pad, your partner's body nestled close in bed), attention to good posture and body mechanics, and sleeping on a firm mattress. Occasionally, pregnancy can aggravate an unknown back problem such as a bony abnormality or disc disease. If your back pain is persistent despite your exercise and heat program, see your physician for help. A wise request would be to have him or her refer you to a physical therapist for additional consultation and treatment.

Save Wear and Tear on Your Back

Approaching everyday tasks with an eye to pregnant body mechanics can also save much wear and tear on your back. The single most stressful situation is when you reach to pick up an object lower than your hips: newspaper, kids' clothes, the can on the bottom shelf, a pet, a child. Most often, people simply bend forward from the waist, scoop up the object, and straighten up. STOP! Even if the object is very light, you are placing excessive strain on your lower back. A long lever arm has been created out of the upper portion of your body with the muscles of the lower back as the fulcrum (stress point). Those softened ligaments are doing

LIFTING

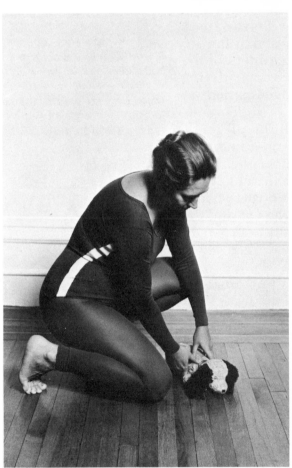

Saves strain on lower back.

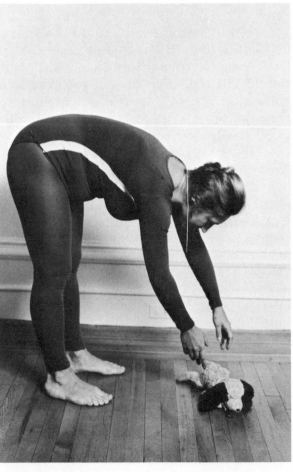

Stresses lower back.

much more work than they were designed for. To eliminate this problem, train yourself to lift using the muscles of your legs for the heavy work:

1. get close to the object;
2. place one foot ahead of the other;
3. bend knees into a squatting position, keeping back straight;
4. bring object close to your body; and
5. straighten legs so you rise up smoothly.

Picking up a toddler is easier if you have the child climb up on a footstool or piece of furniture before you attempt to lift.

Take care of your back while arising from a supine position, too. Your slackened abdominal muscles are of little help in this by the end of pregnancy, so:

1. roll over onto your side,
2. swing legs over the side of the bed while
3. placing hands on bed surface and straightening arms so upper body is elevated,
4. tilt pelvis backward and stand up.

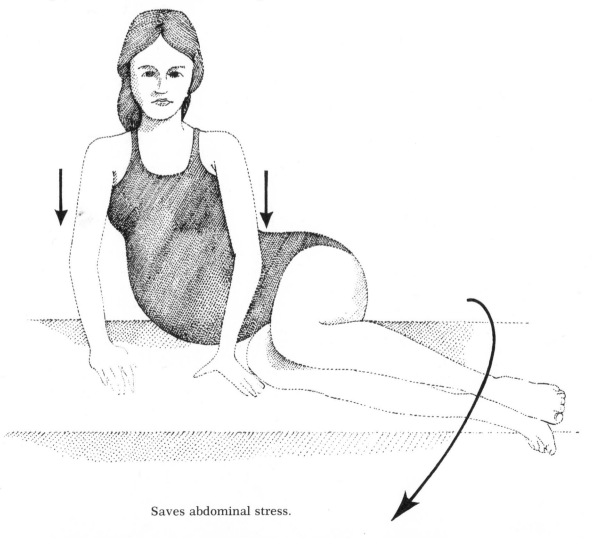

Saves abdominal stress.

I have had chronic low back pain since the birth of my first baby. I was placed flat on my back during the delivery with my legs strapped into stirrups. The baby was "stuck" at the pubic bone (I now realize this was due to my position), and the doctor used forceps to push her under the bone and pull her out. As she was coming through, I heard a cracking sound in my lower back—a cracked coccyx—and I can no longer sleep on my stomach. The pelvic rocking during subsequent pregnancies has helped relieve the pain, but my back always feels tired.

Reverse the procedure when lying down, allowing your body to release gradually into the mattress after you are down. Sudden shifts in body position can tug on the ligaments which work like guy wires to hold the uterus in place. Sharp, momentary pain can shoot up from the groin or the side of the abdomen as the ligaments stretch and then snap back to their customary shape and position.

A final consideration about your back is to make sure you maintain good posture when sitting. A firm pillow or bath towel rolled into a cylindrical shape and tucked snugly between the lower back and the chairback will give extra support to this overworked area. This is especially important for women who sit in chairs for long periods of time at their work, but it also applies when you ride in the car, watch television, sew, go out for dinner, or attend a concert, movie, or theatre production. Today's oversized tote bags can easily accommodate your pillow or towel so you can keep your back from becoming unnecessarily fatigued wherever you go! An upright posture also makes room for normal breathing and digestion to take place, reducing your difficulties with the shortness of breath and heartburn that seem to plague so many pregnant women.

Go for Loose-Fitting Clothes

Other changes during pregnancy require different types of comfort measures. Probably the best-known of these are loose-fitting clothes to allow room for your expanding abdomen. But what of your feet? They need room to expand, too, especially in late pregnancy when you may have a considerable amount of normal swelling throughout your body. When buying or making maternity clothing and footwear, you should also know that pregnant women often seem to be much warmer than others in a room. Probably this is due to the dramatically expanded blood volume (about 50 percent above nonpregnant levels in most women) and generally higher rates of metabolic activity during pregnancy.

So, when selecting clothes, look for soft, absorbent fabrics that breathe rather than tightly woven synthetics that trap body heat. Choose flat sandals whenever possible for wearing indoors instead of heavy boots. Keeping the foot in close contact with the ground helps you maintain your balance, and a minimum of heel allows your calf muscles to work normally instead of being tightened into a knot all day. Your legs, after all, work much harder because of your increased weight even if your daily routine remains the same.

Along the lines of leg and foot care, you may find

support panty hose (*never* hose which requires garters!) a boon. A soak in the tub at the end of the day always feels good, but consider a tub break at midday if you can. Even a brief foot bath is refreshing—especially if you have a whirlpool fixture for your tub. Use a footstool whenever possible. If swelling bothers you, lie down for 10 to 15 minutes three or four times a day with your legs elevated above your hips to allow the blood pooled in your feet and ankles to drain back to your heart.

If your rings feel too tight on your fingers, simply remove them.

Investing in bras which provide real support for your heavier and fuller breasts makes sense for most women. Special maternity bras are not needed, but by the sixth month or so, you will probably have grown a cup size and maybe two to four inches around. If you plan to wear nursing bras (which feature flaps to bare the nipple without adjusting the over-the-shoulder strap), you will still be able to wear those larger-sized bras after you wean your baby. Your expanded rib cage gradually diminishes in size during the year after your baby is born, so you can anticipate being back to your original size by the time your baby takes that first step.

Look for Ways to Conserve Your Energy

The last few weeks of pregnancy move at a more deliberate pace. As one mother commented, "You feel full in all directions. You understand why flights of stairs have landings. You begin to appreciate ways of conserving energy. You are grateful to others for all the routine chores they volunteer to do for you. You prize quiet times with your mate, marveling at the vigorous antics of your unborn child." Specific ways to check fatigue include:

1. Limit unimportant appointments, meetings, and social obligations. There will be plenty of time to participate in community life after you and your baby have had time to get accustomed to one another.
2. Become acquainted with other women in your area who can be motherhood colleagues. If you are leaving a job which has taken you away from home most of the time, it is important to maintain contact with people. No matter how much you are enjoying pregnancy, there will be times when you need a chance to talk to another adult. Find out where mothers congregate (the park, the laundromat, the neighborhood center) and inquire if there is a child-care co-op in operation. By agreeing to

care for other mothers' children in return for their watching yours, you can plan rest periods for yourself and expand your circle of colleagues quite quickly.

3. Plan your day to include at least a half hour of complete rest (not reading, watching television, or knitting) in midafternoon. This is an important habit to cultivate because in the early weeks postpartum, resting for short periods is the rule, not the exception.

4. Pressure on your bladder may awaken you several times in the night, or the baby's movements may be so strong as to prevent you from falling asleep as soon as you go to bed, or the upward pressure of the uterus on your diaphragm may make you feel uncomfortably short of breath. Explore positions and aids to relaxation, so that even if sleep does not come right away or is interrupted, your muscles are in repose. Many mothers find sleeping easier with a wedge of foam at their backs (ask for a medical wedge at a shop which cuts and covers pillows and mattresses to order) or with extra pillows under their abdomen, between the legs, and tucked behind the lower back. All of these items may be useful during labor, as well, when the mother's comfort and ability to relax are of paramount importance.

5. Develop relaxation skills (see next chapter) so you can take best advantage of the rest periods you have.

The Ever-Useful Tailor Sit Position

A final comfort measure for pregnancy that will be of value to you for years to come is the Tailor Sit Position. Most of us have been trained to sit in chairs ever since we could

TAILOR SITTING

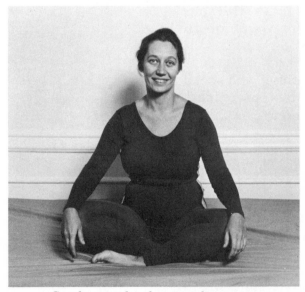

Gently stretches leg muscles.

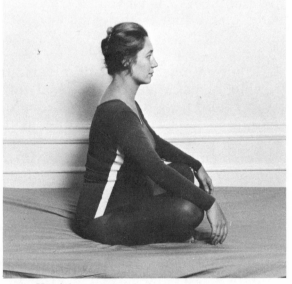

Keep back straight.

be propped in a high chair. But evidence from Asian and Middle Eastern cultures suggests that varicose veins of the legs and of the anus (hemorrhoids) can be prevented by floor sitting and squatting.

You can Tailor Sit almost anywhere while doing many ordinary tasks. All you need is room to cross your legs, keeping them at hip level. Once you get used to it, the position even becomes comfortable for eating. Your small children will enjoy picnic meals with you if you spread a cloth on the floor and have everyone sit around it. Or, try serving dinner for just yourself and your husband in the living room—with you using the cocktail table. Try dining out at Japanese restaurants which feature traditional floor seating. Remind yourself to keep your shoulders back while Tailor Sitting so you don't get weary in the lower back. A variation of the crossed legs position is to extend legs straight in front of you. This position allows you to rotate your feet and ankles if they begin to tingle.

In addition to promoting better circulation in your legs, Tailor Sitting gently stretches the muscles of your inner thigh. Your pushing efforts during the second stage of labor will be enhanced by this extra flexibility. Another distinct advantage of sitting with legs spread wide rather than demurely crossed at the ankle is that you create a convenient resting place for your swelling middle. Placing a bed pillow under your abdomen while Tailor Sitting often relieves the heaviness and downward pressure that accompany the last few weeks of pregnancy.

Conditioning Birth Muscles

Your choice of position for giving birth and your ability to cooperate with your body during the strong expulsive contractions that bring forth your baby depend on many factors. Your nutrition, type of childbirth education, birth expectations, and the unique spatial relationships between your pelvis and the size and position of your baby are all important. Understanding the dynamics of the pushing process explains why two exercises to condition the birth muscles, Squatting and Kegels, are also worth perfecting.

By the time you are about to begin labor, the pregnancy hormones have loosened and relaxed the ligaments which join your pelvic bones. The baby's presenting part (that part of the body which is coming first through the birth canal, usually the head, but in five percent of cases, the buttocks or breech) has settled into the pelvic cavity. During one of your early prenatal appointments, the midwife or doctor has examined you internally to determine the size and shape of your pelvis. If you think of the pelvis as a bony bucket, the wider, upper rim is called the inlet. The outlet is formed at the smaller, lower end where the bones end and the soft tissues of the vagina and surrounding perineum (pelvic floor) begin. The connections between the bones form the sacroiliac joints in the lower back and the pubis in the front. Because these joints have softened during pregnancy, they are spread apart slightly as the baby emerges from your body. This phenomenon, coupled with the softness of the baby's skull bones at birth, make it possible for the overwhelming majority of babies to be propelled through the birth canal by the involuntary contractions of the uterus and abdominal muscles.

As labor progresses, the longitudinal muscles of the uterus gradually pull on the cervix, or neck of the womb, thinning it and drawing it upward into the uterine wall. With each contraction, these long muscle fibers shorten a bit behind the baby, so the presenting part is moved farther and farther down in the pelvis toward the outlet. In a normal labor, progress is determined by feeling the cervix to check its effacement (thinning) and dilatation (degree of open-

PROGRESS IN LABOR

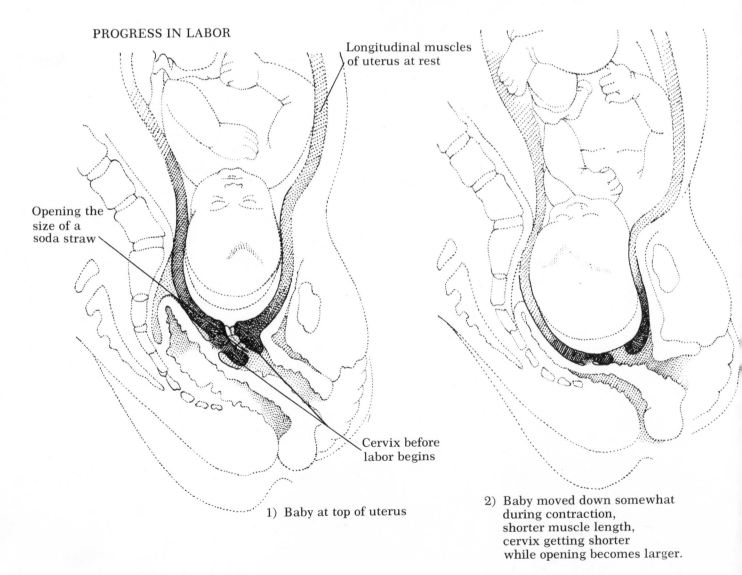

Longitudinal muscles of uterus at rest

Opening the size of a soda straw

Cervix before labor begins

1) Baby at top of uterus

2) Baby moved down somewhat during contraction, shorter muscle length, cervix getting shorter while opening becomes larger.

ness) and by feeling how far into the pelvis the presenting part has descended (station). Once the cervix is out of the way, the downward force of the uterine contractions meets with little resistance from soft maternal tissues and the baby is pushed out the short distance remaining. The action of the uterus is regulated by a naturally secreted hormone, oxytocin, which causes the uterine muscles to contract independently of the mother's will. The objective of exercise for the birth muscles is to allow the baby to be pushed from your body in as gentle and unhurried a manner as possible.

Hard to Devise a Worse Birth Position Than Standard One in United States

The standard birth position in this country, the lithotomy position, places undue stress on mother and baby and contributes to the high rate of surgical intervention in

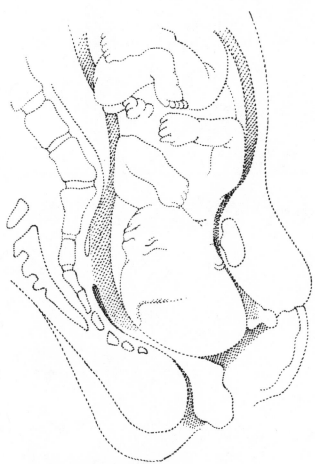

3) Beginning second stage
   Cervix is completely taken up into uterine wall.
   Head is coming into vagina (birth canal).
   Opening is now large enough to allow baby's head
   (usually 10 cm.) through.

For my first labor, I was on my side for the first stage of labor and on my back for the second stage. I had an episiotomy with a tear through the rectal sphincter and up into the body of the rectum. For my third labor, I was on my hands and knees all the way and had only a very minor tear with no episiotomy. What a difference there was in terms of comfort!

what should be spontaneous births. From the physical therapist's point of view, it would be difficult to devise a birth position more incompatible with physiology. Requiring the mother to lie flat on her back with her legs strapped high and wide into stirrups, even when she is awake and unmedicated, is a common cause of chronic back problems, exaggerated separation of the abdominal muscles (*diastasis recti*), and extensive cutting and repair of the skin and muscles which comprise the pelvic floor (episiotomy).

Recent studies by Dr. Roberto Caldeyro-Barcia, president of the International Federation of Obstetricians and Gynecologists, have shown that lying flat on your back also reduces the pelvic outlet to its smallest diameter, thus creating a "closed door" through which the baby is being pushed. The weight of the heavy uterus rests on the large blood vessels which return blood from the legs, reducing the return of blood to the mother's heart and ultimately reduc-

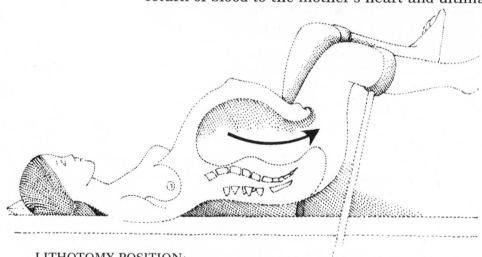

LITHOTOMY POSITION:
buttocks lift up, works against normal uterine forces.

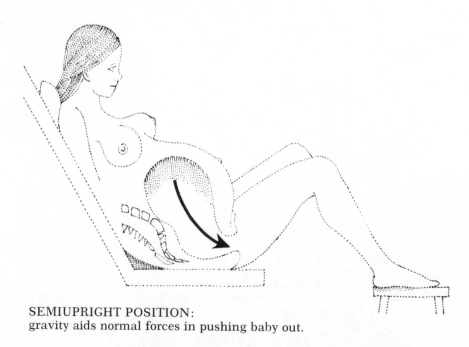

SEMIUPRIGHT POSITION:
gravity aids normal forces in pushing baby out.

ing the supply of blood to the baby. Additionally, the strength of the contractions may lift the mother's hips off the table, so she ends up trying to push the baby not down and out, but up toward the ceiling.

In many other cultures throughout history, women frequently assume a squatting position for birth. In this position, the pelvic outlet is at its widest, the birth canal is shortened, and the uterus is assisted by gravity so contractions are more efficient. It is unlikely that your hospital birth attendants will encourage you to assume the full squatting position—primarily because they cannot see what is happening—but a modified squat, with the mother propped at a 45-degree angle, can usually be arranged.

Many women can squat like a toddler without difficulty. Remember to keep your heels flat when you squat to obtain the most stretch in your legs from doing the exercise. It is also a good idea to bend forward slightly at the waist before you go down to keep your balance. Obviously, squatting to pick things up not only saves your back from strain, but also increases the flexibility of your inner thigh muscles. It is also the most comfortable way to reach something lower than your hips, especially toward the end of pregnancy when you may find your abdomen so enlarged that bending over is virtually impossible.

The squatting practice is a bonus during lovemaking, too. I can get much closer to my husband even though my belly is expanded!

SQUATTING

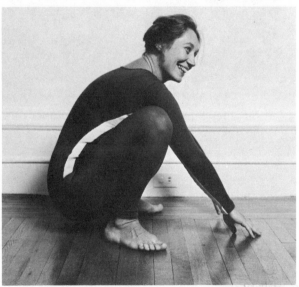

Full squat: feet flat, knees behind shoulders.

If you have trouble getting down into a full Squat, you may need to stretch your hip ligaments and inner thigh muscles gradually. The Modified Squat exercise is done with a partner. Sit on the floor, leaning back toward the wall on pillows or cushions at a 45-degree angle. Make sure your back is comfortable and supported firmly. Draw your knees up as close to your shoulders as possible, then slide forearms under to support legs and keep them off the floor. Spread your legs as far apart as you can. Next, have your partner place his/her hands just above the knees on the inner thigh and *gently, steadily* ease them a bit farther apart. Your partner should stop when you feel a stretch in your inner thigh and groin, then sustain the pressure for 15 seconds. You may then release your legs completely, shake them out on the floor in front of you, then repeat the entire sequence two or three times. The Modified Squat should be done once a day from early pregnancy until you can move easily into the full Squat. The full Squat, if comfortable, can be incorporated into your everyday patterns of doing things for the remainder of your pregnancy.

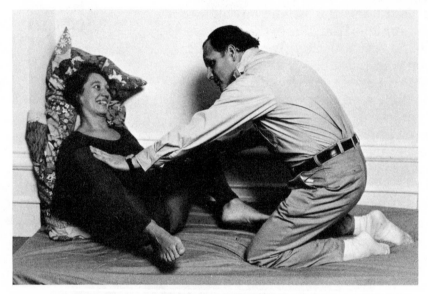

Modified Squat: gently stretching inner thighs; comfortable birth position.

Preventing Episiotomy

A second set of exercises are extremely important both during birth and for regaining muscle tone postpartum. The pregnancy hormones have allowed the soft tissues and muscles of the pelvic floor to relax in preparation for the stretching they will undergo as the baby passes through. Consciously releasing the pelvic floor while pushing contractions are in progress reduces trauma to maternal tissues and increases your chances of giving birth without an episiotomy.

The pelvic floor is comprised of several sheets of muscle suspended like a hammock beneath the uterus from the pubic bone in front to the coccyx (tailbone) in back. The pelvic floor has three openings—to urethra, vagina, and rectum—over which you have voluntary control. Another name for the pelvic floor muscle group is the pubococcygeal, or PC, muscle, so named because of its suspension points. The pelvic floor supports all your internal organs, including uterus, bladder, and bowel, so careful attention to it greatly reduces your chances of gynecological problems later in life.

The series of exercises recommended for the pelvic floor were originated by Dr. Arnold Kegel of UCLA, a well-known specialist in surgical repair of prolapsed (fallen) uteri, prolapsed bladders, and flabby vaginas. Realiz-

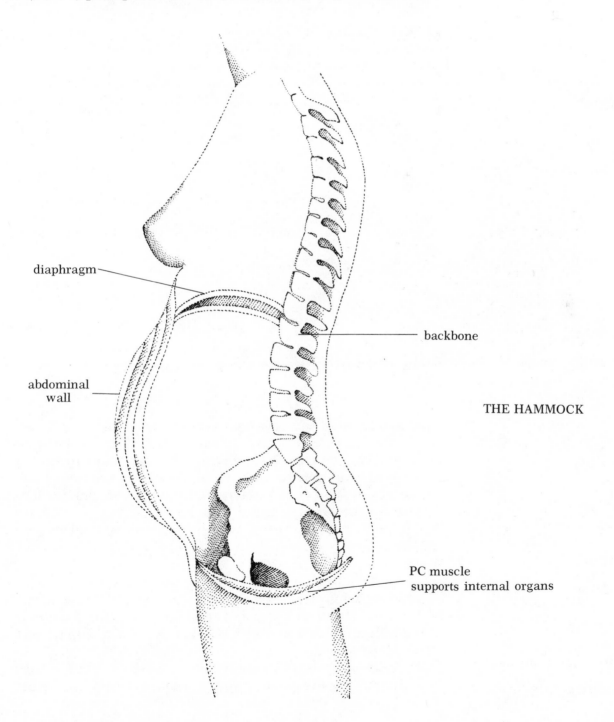

diaphragm

backbone

abdominal
wall

THE HAMMOCK

PC muscle
supports internal organs

Kegel Exercise Muscles

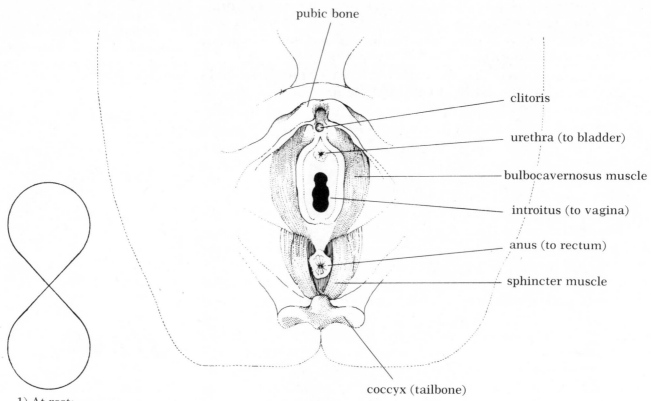

pubic bone

clitoris

urethra (to bladder)

bulbocavernosus muscle

introitus (to vagina)

anus (to rectum)

sphincter muscle

coccyx (tailbone)

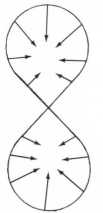

1) At rest:
   forms figure 8
   around urethra,
   vagina, and anus.

2) Squeeze in
   during Kegel.

Note: Kegel exercise:
   pulling in all parts
   of the figure 8,
   making it smaller.

The Hammock:
Muscles supporting the pelvic floor are suspended between
pubic bone and coccyx.

ing that most of the surgery he performed could be avoided if women learned how to take care of the PC muscle during pregnancy, he authored many articles about restitution of tone and function to the pelvic floor by exercise alone. Because of his pioneering work in the field, pelvic floor exercises are often referred to as Kegels.

The first steps toward keeping your pelvic floor in good shape are:

1. Find the muscle. The next time you are sitting on the toilet urinating, try to slow down or stop the flow of the urine. If you can stop and start it several times without difficulty, begin the Elevator exercise; otherwise, follow step 2.

2. Apply some lubricating jelly (such as K-Y jelly) to your finger, then insert into your vagina. Squeeze the finger

tightly as though trying to hold back a bowel movement and the flow of urine. You'll feel a tightening down on the finger in the vagina since all the muscle fibers of the pelvic floor are connected. Now that you've identified the muscle contraction, go on to Kegels.

Try the Elevator Concept

Imagine that your pelvic floor is a slow, flat, freight elevator with a heavy load, and it has just closed its doors on the first floor. You slowly start to tighten the muscles and the elevator moves up to the second floor. You tighten a little more and move to the third floor—hold tight for five full seconds and then move up to the fourth floor. Now you discover you can't unload yet so you *slowly* start down to the third floor as you relax just slightly. Gradually go to the second, then the first floor. But now you find out you can unload in the basement, so you have to go down one more, and you are actually bulging the muscles outward a little as you sink below the starting level. Repeat the exercise five times and do it slowly at least ten times a day for a total of 50 times.

The bulging or opening up will become an unconscious accompaniment to bearing down with the second-stage contractions of birth. Sometimes, untrained women actually tighten the pelvic floor during birth rather than releasing, so with practice you can learn good control and good conscious relaxation of these muscles. This will allow you to avoid the unconscious tightening during birth. Dr. Robert Bradley, author of *Husband-Coached Childbirth* (New York: Harper and Row, 1974), calls this the "open door policy" of childbirth.

Communication Exercise. You need your partner for this exercise. After intercourse, you can try tightening and relaxing your PC muscle on your man's penis. He can keep track of your increasing strength.

Red Light Exercise. Every time you see a red light while driving (traffic light, taillight), do two pelvic-floor-tightening contractions.

The goal of the exercise is to keep good tone and support for the pelvic organs and to teach you how to relax the muscle during the birth of the baby. The exercise will not automatically prevent you from having an episiotomy. The muscles, skin, and vaginal walls were all expertly designed to stretch enough to give birth, but there is much controversy about whether a woman should also have an incision through the skin and muscle to enlarge the vaginal outlet for birth, thus speeding the second stage of labor. Most physicians trained in this country believe the incision

I found that by practicing Kegels in front of the mirror I had a much better idea of what I was doing. It also helped to practice pushing this way—I could see when my perineum was bulging and I was pushing correctly.

should be made early to prevent tearing, yet midwives and doctors in other countries rarely find episiotomy necessary.

If an episiotomy seems necessary in your case, you should discuss your preference for a "pressure" episiotomy, done very late in the second stage without anesthetic, with your birth attendant. Nature provides numbness to the entire perineum at the height of each pushing contraction due to the pressure of the baby's head on the tissues, so you will not feel the incision, but you do feel the baby come through. Many women look forward to this moment as the climax of many hours of labor. They describe the sensation as being comparable to the release of orgasm after the buildup of physical stimulation and emotional energy. It is a supreme gratification which they speak of joyously for years afterward.

Endurance

Although the exercises we have discussed so far will improve muscular strength and flexibility, they contribute nothing to heart and lung efficiency, commonly termed endurance.

Exercises to improve endurance are called aerobic exercises. By continuing an activity for a sufficiently long period of time, you create a demand in your body for oxygen. Repeating the activity, such as brisk walking or jogging, at least three times a week for approximately 20 to 30 minutes causes changes in your heart and lungs which improve your body's efficiency in utilizing oxygen—termed conditioning. It results in a significant improvement in your ability to perform prolonged physical work.

In his book, *The New Aerobics* (New York: M. Evans and Co., 1970), Dr. Kenneth H. Cooper describes childbirth as "the greatest challenge the average woman faces during her life."

During the first six months of your pregnancy, your conditioning program can start with walking and then include any of the graduated programs included in *Aerobics for Women*, written by Mildred and Kenneth Cooper (New York: M. Evans and Co., 1972), such as swimming, cycling, tennis, cross-country skiing, walking, or jogging. After the sixth month, most women are more comfortable with activities that don't require moving their additional body weight, such as riding a stationary bicycle or swimming. Since this form of exercise is the most beneficial in terms of overall health for the time in your life when you are not pregnant, it would be worthwhile to read Cooper's book and also get your partner involved (the first book includes charts for men).

I found that walking a mile or two every day during the first two pregnancies kept me feeling energetic. During my third pregnancy, I didn't make a big effort to get out and walk, and I gained ten extra pounds. All the babies were over nine pounds, but it has taken longer to return to my normal weight this time.

Postpartum

Ideally, each woman who has given birth should have at least a one-hour session with a physical therapist to plan and implement an individual exercise program. This program would start within 24 hours after the birth and would be continued for approximately the next nine months. This should take into consideration the woman's prepregnancy physical condition and be arranged to achieve either that state or a goal of an improved fitness level.

Many of the major physiological changes of pregnancy have reverted back to the baseline within six to eight weeks, but the more subtle changes, such as ligamentous loosening, take a longer period. Many popular pamphlets and books on pregnancy give only token references to these changes and describe rather vigorous exercises that could contribute to additional back and pelvic pain. Many other women simply return to daily activities, expecting their muscles to revert back to shape. Unfortunately "Tincture of Time" will do little to tone and increase strength without specific properly graduated exercise.

The following exercises would be a reasonable postpartum recovery program for a woman who had been healthy before and during pregnancy. Be sure you mention to your physician or midwife that you are planning to begin exercises, so that he or she can inform you of any circumstances that might affect your plan. Always heed what your body is telling you—pain means something is wrong, either the wrong position, exercising too fast, or progressing in the sequence too quickly. If you are certain that you have followed the directions and are using good body mechanics throughout the day and you still have pain with specific movements, then consult your physician once more.

Reconditioning the Pelvic Floor

The exercises you practiced during pregnancy to strengthen and consciously release the pelvic floor muscles will now be the basis of your first postpartum exercise. This can and should be started as soon after the birth as you think of it.

If you had an episiotomy, then start slowly to tighten the vaginal muscles while the local anesthetic (injected like novocaine for dental work so that you wouldn't feel the stitches being put in) is still wearing off. Don't be afraid of disturbing the stitches; you are actually shortening the muscles and pulling the incision closer together. This exercise will increase the circulation and remove waste products in the bloodstream as it brings in fresh blood and

I had a pressure episiotomy with my second pregnancy. I had little discomfort with it compared to the first episiotomy, after which I couldn't sit for weeks. Could Kegels have helped?

nutrients to aid healing. As the anesthetic wears off, you may be given a small ice pack for your perineum, or after 48 hours, warm soaks and/or a rubber glove filled with warm water and covered with a warm damp washcloth may be helpful.

Gradually contract your muscles a little bit tighter for one or two more seconds until you are eventually able to do the Elevator exercise again. During the first few days you may be having difficulty even feeling if you have the right muscles moving, but don't give up. You will be able to pace yourself on this exercise via your own comfort.

If you didn't need an episiotomy, you will still need to do this exercise quite regularly. After the stretching of all the muscle fibers and skin, you should begin immediately to shorten them again even before you get up from the position you were in during birth. Try to remember to contract these muscles before you stand or sit down to avoid the feeling of having something give way.

Many other cultures recognize the need for restoration of this muscle group after birth. If it is allowed to remain loose and weak, the uterus may tip or actually sink partway down the vagina. Other problems such as dribbling of urine when you cough or laugh (stress incontinence) can occur.

Women in this country have undergone countless gynecological surgeries for repair of these problems, many of which could have been prevented in the first place. Arnold Kegel, one of the few researchers in this area, documented remarkable success in avoiding surgery and, if it was necessary, recovery from it by teaching women pelvic floor (Kegel) exercises.

Reconditioning the Abdomen

You may have expected a somewhat different appearance to your belly right after the birth. It is a very common idea that you will reach down right after your baby is born and put your hand on your belly—the belly you had before you were pregnant. It is probably closer to the size when you were five months pregnant, plus you're now missing the enlarged uterus that gave the illusion of taut muscles.

The truth is that you have to embark on an active program of abdominal strengthening that is well planned and paced. A crash diet and vigorous exercise have only negative effects. It was mentioned before but deserves repetition—the hormones that loosened all the ligaments and connective tissue prior to the birth are still present in your body, and the changes in your ligaments, joints, and muscles will take several months to occur. It is essential that you use good body mechanics, avoid improper lifting or straining, and approach exercise as a therapeutic tool.

Follow this sequence:

Day 1. While lying on your back, blow all your air out through your lips as though you are blowing out a candle, only keep exhaling slowly and steadily until you can't possibly continue. Your abdominal muscles will be tightening and pulling in. Now, keep them contracted tightly while you inhale and exhale through your nose slowly (but not as deeply as the first time) five times. Repeat this exercise five times the first day.

Day 2. Lying on your back with your knees bent, tighten and draw in your belly muscles. While keeping them tight, do your Pelvic Tilt as you practiced before the birth. Your buttocks are tightened as you push your low back into the floor. Hold tight for a full count of five out loud and then slowly relax first your buttocks, then your abdominals, then relax the tilt. Repeat five times, three times a day.

Day 3. Repeat the above exercise, but this time add lifting your head up at the same time that you are holding the tilt and counting out loud for five full seconds. Repeat five times, two times a day.

Now stop exercising for a few minutes and evaluate how your abdominal wall has survived the past nine months. The abdominal muscles are really four sets of muscles that surround your abdomen much as a large girdle with four-way stretch would.

A line is formed of thick connective tissue down the middle of your abdomen, and this may have darkened during your pregnancy. The line is where most of your abdominal muscles are attached to your ribs and pelvis. This strip of thick tissue is stretched during pregnancy and the abdominal muscles may actually separate. This is called *diastasis recti.* If the separation is large or allowed to continue untreated you will have permanent weakening of your abdominal wall with its secondary effects of low back discomfort and altered body mechanics.

To check for *diastasis recti,* repeat the same exercise you just did and put your fingers on this line right around your navel. If you can fit more than two fingers in the space between the bands of muscle then you must do the following exercise for ten repetitions at least five times a day.

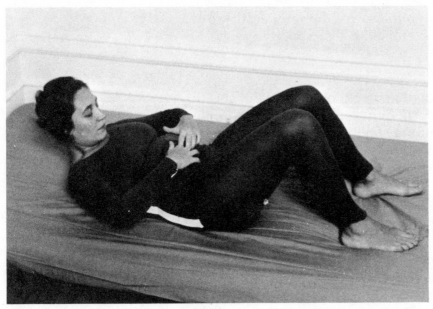

Checking for separated abdominal wall (*diastasis recti*).

ABDOMINAL WALL

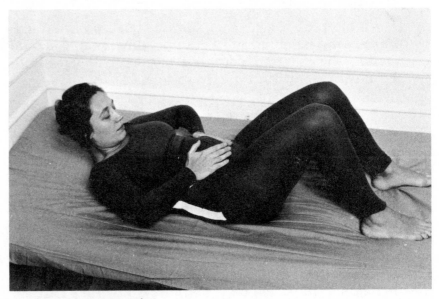

Correcting separation.

Special Exercise for *Diastasis Recti*

Lying on your back with knees bent, put your hands on each side of the abdomen. Take in a deep breath, and as you exhale, lift your head up (and later your shoulders); at the same time, gently push the underlying muscles together toward the midline. Lie back slowly. If you are faithful with doing the exercise, the gap should return to the normal ½ inch within a week or so. This should be accomplished before you progress with the rest of the exercise.

Days 4 and 5. You should still be doing your Pelvic Tilt and lifting up your head as you exhale and count out loud to five. As soon as this feels more comfortable, try lifting your shoulders off the floor and bring your chin down to your chest.

By today (fourth or fifth), try your Pelvic Tilt while standing as you did during pregnancy. If it feels com-

DIASTASIS RECTI

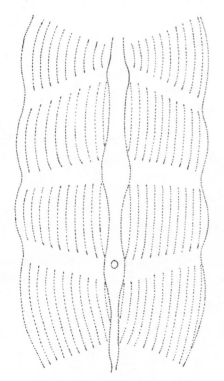

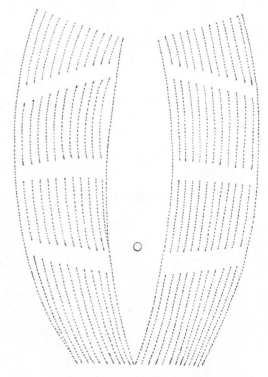

Abdominal muscles in nonpregnant woman

The recti muscles can separate as a zipper opens under stress, weakening the abdominal wall. Elizabeth Noble, R.P.T., originated this "zipper concept," and it is discussed fully in her book, *Essential Exercises for the Childbearing Year*, Boston: Houghton Mifflin Co., 1976.

fortable, proceed on with the sequence. You may have many variables in the speed of the progression. If an exercise produces unusual soreness or discomfort, then spend a few more days on the preceding exercise.

Day 6. Today, start doing your Pelvic Tilt on all fours and remember to tighten your abdomen and, as best you can, your buttocks. You'll remember, from doing this exercise during pregnancy, that it is more difficult to contract your buttocks in this position. Maintain the tucked-in position for five to six seconds and relax. Repeat 15 times. Increase the number of repetitions and, if possible, repeat three times a day over the next week.

Day 14. By approximately two weeks after you start your program, you should be ready to start a program of Modified Sit-ups. There are several principles to follow for sit-ups that should be applied for this group of exercises.

1. Always keep your knees bent and feet flat on floor; never exercise with your legs straight. This would arch your back and strain it besides allowing the substitution of other muscle groups.
2. Always exhale as you do the movement to prevent straining; never hold your breath. A good reminder to breathe is if you say, *out loud*, one, one thousand, two, one thousand, three, one thousand, four, one thousand, five, one thousand, and so on.
3. Don't hook your feet under any object or let anyone stabilize your legs for you, since this also would allow muscle substitution.
4. It's only necessary to sit up two-thirds of the way. The sequence can be explained and the number of repetitions should be five to ten, but the frequency and speed of the progression will have to be individual. It may vary from several weeks to several months. The resistance to your abdominal muscles is provided by how your arms are placed.

1st Position: The easiest position is with your arms straight in front of you reaching for your knees as you do a partial sit-up. Variation: Alternate sitting up this way with reaching both arms to one side of your knees, then the other side. This diagonal sit-up will strengthen the side abdominal muscles.

2nd Position: The next position of increasing difficulty is with your arms folded across your chest. Repeat both variations.

3rd Position: Put your hands behind your head as you do the sit-ups and turn your upper body for a variation of sideways sit-up.

An optional exercise for your buttocks would include the early tightening along with your Pelvic Tilt and then later, while lying on your stomach, you can alternate lifting your thigh up off the floor while keeping your knee bent. Hold it up in the air for a count of five and only do one leg at a time. If you have any feeling of strain in your lower back, discontinue this exercise.

The preceding program is geared to restoring tone and muscle strength. It works best if combined with a well-balanced diet and adequate protein intake. The postpartum period is no time for extreme reducing diets. Fatigue is very common and frequent rest must be obtained whenever the demands of your baby allow it. If necessary, call on friends, family, or hired help for housekeeping chores so that you have adequate time for your own and your baby's health and well-being.

Cesarean Birth

If you had your baby via surgery rather than a vaginal birth, then there are essential differences in your postpartum recovery and rehabilitation. Although most of this type of surgery is done with regional anesthesia (where the mother is numb from the rib cage down), she is awake and draped so she can't see the surgery but will be able to see the baby right after it is born. Occasionally general anesthesia (mother is asleep) is necessary.

In the latter case, your lungs need immediate reexpansion. As soon as you awaken, start taking about ten slow, very deep breaths so that your ribs expand at the bottom. Once you are out of the recovery room, continue to do the deep breathing exercise about once an hour, and also do your diaphragmatic breathing. These breathing exercises will help loosen any phlegm or mucus that collects in your lungs during the surgery. Since it's important to get rid of this phlegm to prevent pneumonia, take in a deep breath, hold your incision, and "huff." This "huff" is not quite as uncomfortable as a cough and if you get in enough air first and then breathe a short, sharp "ha" you should be able to expel the mucus. The incision will be uncomfortable, but don't worry about the stitches, they're as strong now as they'll ever be.

Since you will be helped out of bed the next day, start preparing as soon as possible.

Day 1. a. Do a lot of slow, large, ankle circles.

b. Push your legs down into the bed very hard so that the knees stiffen and your buttocks are pinched tight together.

c. Start pelvic floor tightening. Even though you didn't have the vaginal stretching, those muscles were still strained during pregnancy and need additional postpartum strengthening.

d. Slowly bend and straighten knees, one at a time.

Body Mechanics in Bed. Turning from side to side may be difficult, but frequent position changes will help to expel painful gas collections. If you want to turn to the left, bend only your right knee, then bring the right knee over the left leg *at the same time* as you turn your upper body and reach to the left with your right arm. This is called log rolling and eliminates twisting the area of your incision. Also try exhaling as you turn—a moan or groan is fine—just don't hold your breath. Once you are on your side, do some Pelvic Tilts and some pelvic floor exercises to help stimulate return of your bowel and bladder functions.

Someone will help you to your feet soon. If you have time, review the proper method above. Once you're on your feet try to stand tall with good posture. If you bend forward over your incision, your lungs and your intestines are cramped for room.

Day 2. Start slow abdominal tightening as you exhale. This will be difficult to do, but ask your coach to help you with encouragement, because an increase in circulation from exercise will aid the healing of the incision while the contraction of the muscle actually draws the ends closer together.

Days 2 to 5. Repeat the abdominal tightening exercise and by *Day 5,* start adding the Pelvic Tilt and pick up the program in the same sequence as described for the vaginal birth. You will proceed *very slowly* and pace yourself on a day-to-day basis—you should probably expect to double the number of days spent with each step in the sequence. Postpone the exercise until you see your doctor if it causes you any discomfort.

Since both pregnancy and the months after birth are times of tremendous change, these exercises should start you thinking about the natural beauty of your body and its awesome capabilities.

Chart of Exercises Postpartum

	Cardiovascular	Abdominals	Pelvic Floor
Day 1		Pull in belly muscles and hold tight for gradually more seconds.	Start immediately to attempt to rediscover this muscle connection.
Day 2		Pelvic Tilt while on your back.	Continue to extend length of holding it tight.
Day 3		Check for *diastasis recti* while lifting head during Pelvic Tilt.	Increase frequency and lengthen tightening.
Days 4, 5, and 6		Pelvic Tilt while standing up plus continue lifting head while doing Pelvic Tilt.	Continue as above.
Day 7	Begin walking program.	Pelvic Tilt on all fours, increase frequency.	Continue as above.
Day 14	Continue walking program.	Half sit-up with arms forward.	Gradually start "Communication Exercise."
Day 30	Return to aerobic sports or a conditioning program: walking, jogging, biking, swimming.	Full program of sit-ups: arms crossed on chest, doing straight and diagonals. Progress to arms behind head if possible.	Continue pelvic floor contractions daily for the rest of your life.

Recommended Reading

Bradley, Robert, M.D. *Husband-Coached Childbirth.* New York: Harper and Row, 1974.

Cooper, Mildred and Cooper, Kenneth H., M.D. *Aerobics for Women.* New York: M. Evans and Co., 1972.

Cooper, Kenneth, M.D. *The New Aerobics.* New York: M. Evans and Co. (Bantam), 1970.

Fitzhugh, Mabel, R.P.T. *Preparation for Childbirth.* Self-published. San Rafael, California, 1973. Includes exercise chart ($1.25). Send orders to:
Margaret B. Farley, R.P.T.
21 Santa Margarita Drive
San Rafael, CA 94901
Telephone: (415) 456-3143

Heardman, Helen. *Relaxation and Exercise for Natural Childbirth.* 4th ed. Edited by Maria Ebner. New York: Churchill Livingstone, 1975.

*Noble, Elizabeth, R.P.T. *Essential Exercises for the Childbearing Year.* Boston: Houghton Mifflin Co., 1976.

*highly recommended

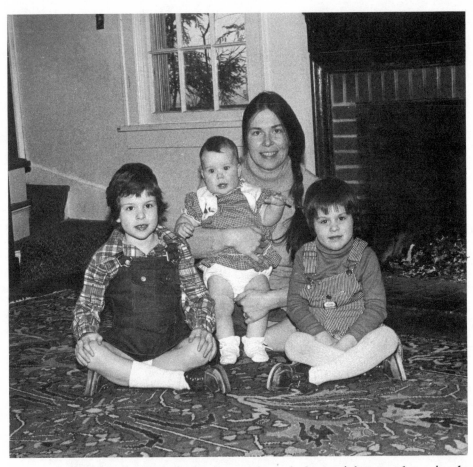

Gail Sforza Brewer is the mother of three girls; two born in the hospital, the last at home when Mrs. Brewer was 32. She attended Wells College and holds B.S. and M.A. degrees in communication from Syracuse University and the University of Wisconsin.

Author of What Every Pregnant Woman Should Know: The Truth About Diets and Drugs in Pregnancy *(New York: Random House, 1977), she is Director of Instructor Training and Certification for the Metropolitan New York Childbirth Education Association. With her husband, Dr. Tom Brewer, she lectures widely and teaches childbirth classes in Croton-on-Hudson, New York.*

4
Cooperative Childbirth: The Woman-Centered Approach by: Gail Sforza Brewer

Every pregnant woman is entitled to an educational program for childrearing that helps her identify and meet her health needs and those of her unborn baby.

Women who conclude that the typical childbirth preparation classes available in their communities do not serve this function find themselves in the position of having to design their own birth education programs. In doing so, they join the ranks of women everywhere who are adopting a self-help approach to women's health matters.

Pregnancy and birth belong in the realm of women's health concerns because they are normal functions for which our bodies are exquisitely adapted. Prevailing medical practice, however, persists in characterizing pregnancy as a deviation from the normal, a "condition" to be treated or managed by disease specialists. This fundamental divergence in outlook amounts to much more than semantics. It governs the care offered to us when we become pregnant.

We experience our pregnancies and births as anxious waits, punctuated by cursory examinations for potential complications, rather than splendid opportunities to learn what we can do for ourselves to bring about the most healthful pregnancies, labors, and offspring possible. Woman-centered childbirth education operates on different assumptions, asks different questions, and returns different solutions to problems than disease-oriented American obstetrics. Woman-centered care is biased in the direction of health maintenance.

Understanding this basic conflict helps firm your resolve as you seek cooperation from institutions and individuals in accomplishing the birth you desire.

Expectations

Regardless of your age, it is realistic to expect childbearing to be one of the most pleasurable and healthful periods in your life. After all, you are an evolutionary creature with all of Nature's past experience on your side! The myriad adaptations taking place in your body are safeguards for mother and baby. Think of them as insurance, if you will, that your baby will be born strong and healthy after an efficient labor that takes place at the appropriate time. Respecting and cooperating with these adaptive mechanisms lays the foundation for a successful

The great thing about going to the Bradley classes was that it was the only place I ever got the feeling that pregnancy was a healthy condition for a woman, and that I would be able to give birth myself without all the drugs and machines. I learned why it was important to eat well and how that was related to my baby's brain development. So, I stopped worrying about the baby being retarded.

Sometimes it seemed that there was so much that had to be learned just to have a baby. We read scores of books, pamphlets, newsletters, and articles. But it was good that we did. This new knowledge made us feel secure and confident in our own abilities to succeed in safely bringing forth a child.

Often we get so caught up in procedures and techniques that we tend to forget that long before obstetricians were invented, women somehow managed to keep the human race well supplied. Obviously, Mother Nature equipped the human female with the capability of giving birth without an attending physician.

79

pregnancy; disregarding them creates conditions for crisis.

Many older women encounter obstetricians who discourage them from planning for a vaginal birth. These physicians claim that a Cesarean section almost always has to be done on older mothers because their "aging" muscles and tissues cannot be expected to withstand the stresses of normal labor. This conclusion may hold true for women who follow these physicians' prescriptions for high-risk pregnancy management: low-salt, low-calorie diets and batteries of biochemical assessment tests. This sort of care produces the very complications of labor the physician ascribes solely to the mother's age. You will find it easier to resist this approach when you know how your body functions during pregnancy.

Your Body/Your Baby

Any rational discussion of human pregnancy must be based on a single essential principle: Mother and baby are one unit. The concept that the needs of mother and baby can be considered independently of each other accounts for much of what is wrong with contemporary prenatal and birth practices. Simply stated, there would be no changes occurring in your body if your baby weren't developing there. Stated another way, your unborn baby is completely dependent on your body systems for survival. Taking care of these body systems is your major health responsibility during pregnancy.

The degree to which your body adjusts healthfully to pregnancy depends extraordinarily on the quality of your daily diet. This point cannot be overemphasized. Any of the intricate developmental phases your baby passes through *in utero* can be disrupted when your diet is inadequate. Without sound nutrition, the old doctor's tale that any complication can occur in any pregnant woman at any time is true! When you eat adequately for your pregnancy, you are secure in the knowledge that you are reducing the risks of complications for yourself and your baby to the absolute minimum. The normal course of pregnancy, birth, and postpartum described subsequently assumes that you are well nourished according to the standards explained in chapter 2.

Early Pregnancy

By the time you first suspect you might be pregnant, two weeks or so after your first missed period, your unborn baby already has passed many decisive milestones in physical development. From a single cell no larger than the dot at the end of this sentence, the baby's body has grown to

When I learned I was pregnant this time, I immediately began taking vitamin supplements and watching that I was eating good foods. I secured good prenatal care and made sure I got 75 to 80 grams of protein a day. I avoided all medications (even for headaches). I gave birth to a 9-pound, 15-ounce baby boy who had an Apgar score of 10 (the highest score a baby can get). He nursed vigorously right from the start. Now at 3½ months, he weighs 17 pounds, and he was fed only on breast milk, no supplements. We (my husband and I) look at him, and inside we beam because we made his birth an accomplishment.

millions of specialized cells organized into the foundations of functional systems. Though but ¼-inch long, the month-old embryo has rudimentary eyes, spinal cord, brain, sense organs, muscles, digestive tract, blood vessels, and a beating heart.

Placenta

Oxygen and nourishment pass from your bloodstream to the baby via the placenta and umbilical cord from the twelfth day of life. The placenta also begins to manufacture female hormones usually produced by your ovaries. During pregnancy the ovaries become dormant; no new eggs are released, probably a natural safeguard for the pregnancy already underway. A sudden rise in the level of female hormones is believed by some researchers to trigger the nausea which can accompany early pregnancy. Some women report success in dealing with nausea by eating small, high-protein snacks frequently throughout the day and whenever they arise during the night. Others find vitamin B_6 helpful. In cases where vomiting becomes severe, medication can sometimes correct the situation.

Quality nutrition is important in early pregnancy to insure optimum implantation of the placenta on the uterine wall. Defects in placental growth and attachment can result in poor transfer of nutrients to the baby, thus compromising the baby's development. In acute cases, the placenta separates from the uterine wall prematurely (before the birth of the baby). This is a life-threatening complication for mother and baby called abruption of the placenta. Abruption results in complete loss of oxygen to the baby and massive hemorrhage for the mother. It is one of the direst emergencies in obstetrics, and, since it results exclusively from malnutrition, you can prevent it completely by eating enough good foods every day of your pregnancy.

Usually the placenta implants high up on the rear wall of the uterus, a protected location well out of the path the baby must travel during birth. If the placenta develops toward the front wall, it is termed an anterior placenta. This does not affect its function in any way, but a woman scheduled for amniocentesis or Cesarean section should make sure the physician has located the placenta to avoid damaging it before the birth of the baby. Occasionally, and for unknown reasons, the placenta grows in the lower segment, next to or even covering the outlet of the uterus, the cervix. This condition is *placenta previa* (the placenta precedes the baby). In order for the baby to be born vaginally, it must first pass through the cervix. When *placenta previa* exists, the extent to which the outlet is blocked

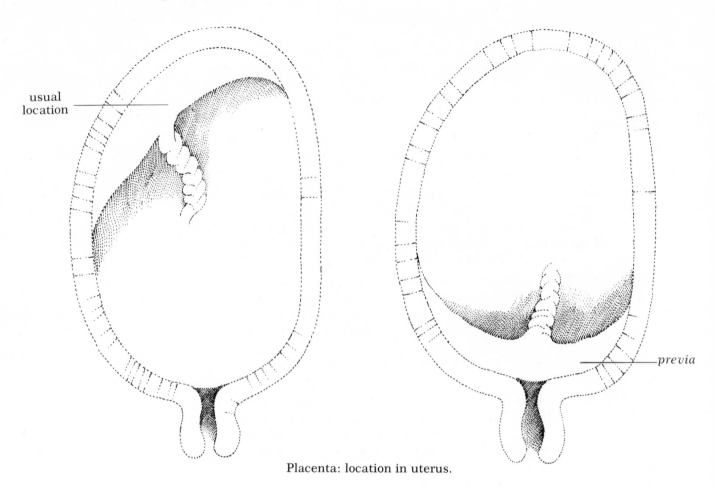

usual
location

previa

Placenta: location in uterus.

determines the manner of birth. If the placenta is low, pressure from the baby's head in the last few weeks may rupture blood vessels in the placenta, causing bright red bleeding. *Placenta previa* is one of many reasons for bleeding in pregnancy. All require that you contact your physician immediately for diagnosis and treatment.

By the time you are ready to give birth, the placenta will be about the size of a dinner plate, approximately one inch thick, weigh one-and-a-half to two pounds and have several hundred yards of contact surface for the transfer of nutrients and waste products between your circulation and that of your baby. The relationship of placental function to increased blood volume and liver function is explained in chapter 2.

Breasts

The growth of the placenta is paralleled in early pregnancy by the growth of your breasts. The placenta facilitates the nutrition of your baby before birth, the breasts afterward. Richard M. Applebaum, M.D., has described breast structure and function very imaginatively in his handbook for nursing mothers, *Abreast of the Times* (7914 SW 104th St., Miami, FL 33156: Self-published, 1969).

I have always thought the cross section of the female breast to be one of the most beautiful diagrams in the medical texts. It has the appearance of a peaceful, well-organized forest. . . . There are 10 to 20 trees or duct systems. Examine one tree. As we look toward the topmost branches we see the leaves (alveoli). The alveoli are secreting gland cells which produce colostrum and later, real milk. Each of these alveoli is surrounded by rubberband-like cells (myoepithelial cells). These cells are activated by a hormone, oxytocin (released when your breasts are stimulated—Ed.), and they literally snap down with positive pressure on the alveoli (like a hand squeezing a sponge) and force milk into the ducts where it travels downward until it reaches the

CROSS SECTION OF THE FEMALE BREAST

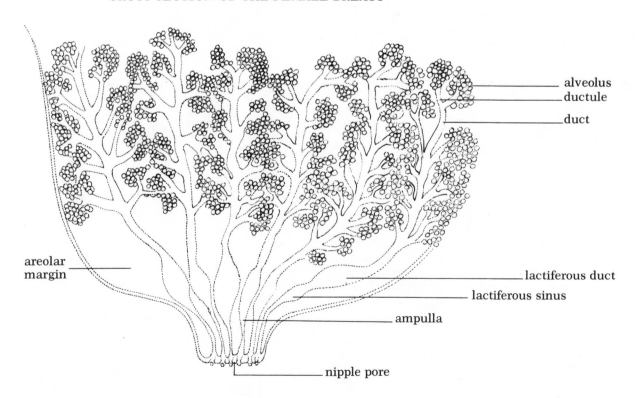

alveolus
ductule
duct

areolar margin

lactiferous duct
lactiferous sinus
ampulla
nipple pore

reservoir (sinus) at the base of the tree. Here, it is held in reserve until it is passed through the roots (nipple openings) of the tree when your baby begins to nurse. The ground or soil covering the roots and reservoirs at the base of our tree is the areolar margin or brown pigmented area of the breast. It is on this margin that the infant sucks.

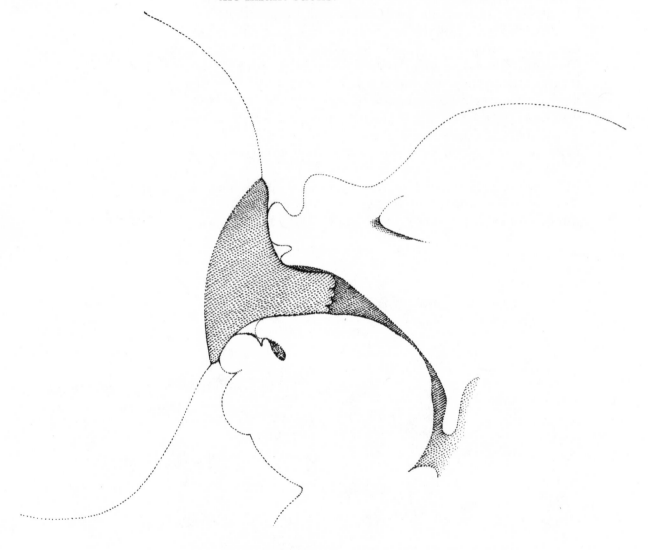

Rising levels of the female hormones, estrogen and progesterone, stimulate the duct system into a period of continuous growth during the first half of pregnancy. Your breasts may feel warmer, more tender, firmer, and fuller as this new tissue proliferates. For many women, these breast changes are the first indication that they are pregnant. By the end of pregnancy and during lactation you will most likely need a bra at least one and perhaps two cup sizes larger than when you started.

Uterus

The most noticeable sign of pregnancy is the dramatic expansion of your uterus to accommodate the growing baby, placenta, amniotic sac, and fluid. During the first few months of pregnancy, though the uterus does enlarge from the size of a peach to that of a grapefruit, you probably won't "show" very much. Several soft organs and tissues surround the uterus in the pelvic basin. In the early months, the swelling uterus first pushes these organs out of the way, making more space for itself within the confines of the bony pelvis. This results in the frequent need to empty your bladder which is so characteristic of early pregnancy.

About the fourth month, the rapidly growing uterus can no longer be cradled in the pelvis. Its topmost margin, the fundus, can be felt rising into the lower abdomen just above the pubic bone. At each subsequent prenatal visit, the midwife, nurse-practitioner, or physician will feel your abdomen and note the height of the fundus. Since many women are not sure exactly when they became pregnant, the fundal measurement is often used to estimate length of gestation and roughly establish a due date.

Monthly increases in size considerably above the normal range may indicate multiple pregnancy. If twins are suspected, the first thing to do is boost your intake of food by at least 500 additional calories and 30 extra grams of protein (this can be done easily by adding the equivalent of one quart of milk to your basic daily diet). There is no truth to the idea that your uterus can only stretch so far and then labor has to begin. As long as you are well nourished for your pregnancy, the uterus will continue to grow regardless of the number of babies you are carrying, and regardless of your age.

The uterus is simply a muscular bag. Like so many other pregnancy adjustments, its pattern of growth depends largely on your nutrition. The uterus enlarges three ways:

1. existing cells lengthen and thicken,
2. new cells form in the uterine wall, and
3. more connective tissue (collagen) is laid down between cells.

Thin, flabby wombs are common in poorly nourished women and are responsible for the higher incidence of prolonged, painful labor these women suffer. The quality of the labor is directly related to the quality of the diet during pregnancy. Especially important for the growth and strength of the uterus are protein and vitamin C, both of which are essential in collagen synthesis.

I ate well and had a great, quick labor.

Most people today are unaware of their body's needs. We've learned to mask body signals in countless ways through the use of painkillers, sedatives, tranquilizers, alcohol, caffeine, nicotine, and drugs of all varieties. In labor it becomes critical that a woman listen to her body. Only she can interpret the message her body conveys.

Every time I was with my parents during my pregnancy, my father would comment on how good I looked and say, "It's those hormones working!"

The strong uterus is much less likely to require artificial stimulation by drugs during labor in order to bring about the birth of the baby. This reduces the chances of the mother requiring medication for pain since her uterine contractions will not be augmented by drugs to the point of becoming unbearably strong. The need for Cesarean section in well-nourished women is also greatly reduced because the uterus functions as it should throughout labor.

Skin

The rush of female hormones into your circulation in early pregnancy is reminiscent of adolescence. Your "teen-age skin" may reappear, blemishes and all, for a few weeks until your body chemistry rights itself. By way of making up for this brief broken-out period, your skin for the rest of pregnancy should take on a blush of health you may not have had since grade school! More blood circulating through your body brings natural color to your cheeks as they fill out from normal water retention (those hormones again!). That extra fluid also diminishes whatever facial expression lines you may have developed as well as fine lines around your eyes. Many older women find that they go through pregnancy looking ten years younger, thanks to these basic skin changes. For that reason alone, it's a marvelous time to be photographed.

Caring for your new, fresh face will probably require less makeup than you might usually use. Plain soap and water are fine cleansing agents unless your skin is dry. Highly perfumed bars may be irritating, especially on your abdomen where the skin is being stretched to the ultimate by the time pregnancy ends. A cream such as Noxzema can soothe dry skin and is easy to use in the shower just by rubbing it into your washcloth. Share your shower time with your mate, and have him do your back—a very relaxing way to end the day, or begin the night.

Speaking of your abdomen, you may be worrying about stretch marks. Women who have an adequate fat intake during pregnancy are much less likely to develop them. If you customarily drink only skim milk and use other fats sparingly, you may find your skin and scalp becoming very dry, overly sensitive, and flaky during pregnancy. The reason: You are probably low in fat-soluble vitamins, particularly vitamin A, which greatly influences the texture of your skin. Switching to whole milk, using more butter or margarine, rediscovering peanut butter, and snacking on other nuts and orange/yellow fruits and vegetables should keep your skin smooth, supple, and moist.

The same principle applies to the lining of your vagina

and the skin of the perineum (pelvic floor). Well-nourished women who give birth in an optimum physiologic position (not flat on the back with legs strapped into stirrups) suffer fewer lacerations of the cervix, vaginal walls, and perineum during birth. The ability of your skin to stretch and gradually slip over the baby's head and shoulders, instead of being surgically widened to facilitate the birth, is conditioned by diet and exercise. (See chapter 3.) Robert A. Bradley, M.D., a pioneer in natural childbirth in the United States, thinks increased circulation of air to the perineum is also important. He comments in *Husband-Coached Childbirth* (New York: Harper and Row, 1975).

> The skin around the vagina is usually brittle and chapped. . .irritated by moist cloth and movement. . . . If you remove the panties, the irritant, you improve the skin. . . . Tight-fitting panty hose are every bit as confining and interfering. Bare bottoms are healthiest.

Another important consideration in caring for your vagina and perineum is the increased glandular activity of normal pregnancy. You may notice heavier vaginal discharge and more perspiration than previously. These changes are normal. If, however, you should develop itching or burning, swelling or redness of tissues, or pain upon urination, you may have an infection. Adequate vitamin A intake prevents minor infections of this sort from blossoming into major complications affecting your bladder, kidneys, and reproductive organs, but you should have the cause of the vaginitis diagnosed and a course of local therapy recommended.

There are two schools of thought about treatments for vaginitis. One is the antibiotic approach; inserting creams or tablets into the vagina to kill the harmful bacteria causing the trouble. The drawback: These medications also kill off healthful bacteria needed to maintain the normal (slightly acidic) vaginal environment. The second approach is restorative; therapies aimed at improving the body's ability to heal itself and prevent further outbreaks. The Vaginal Infections Research Group of the Portland, Oregon Women's Health Clinic shares these tips on preventing vaginitis:

- Wear cotton underpants or none at all.
- Always wipe front to back after a bowel movement.
- Don't share washcloths or towels.
- Avoid chemicals (harsh soaps, perfumed tampons and toilet paper, vaginal deodorants, commercial douches/sprays).

- Eat enough protein and cut sugar and refined foods out of your diet.
- Promote circulation to the genital area by exercise (see chapter 3).
- Never douche during pregnancy (it is possible to force air or fluid into the uterus and abdominal cavity).
- Don't douche routinely, only when necessary for some therapeutic purpose. Douching only washes away the normal mucus which is itself a cleansing agent. This leaves the vagina unprotected and infection is more likely.
- Get enough rest.
- If you develop symptoms, be sure you don't have VD or some other medical problem more serious than a vaginal infection. If you have fever or pain in your lower abdomen, insist on a complete checkup before beginning any treatment.

A final note about your skin: Expect the pigmentation around your nipples to darken and a brownish line to appear running from your pubic bone up to your navel. These areas lighten after pregnancy and, in some cases, return completely to their prepregnancy shade. As you might think, darker-complexioned individuals have more pronounced pregnancy pigmentation than blondes or redheads.

Sleep Needs

As your body adjusts to all these changes in early pregnancy, you may find your needs for sleep vastly increased. Learn to pay attention to your body's messages instead of trying to overcome them. Pregnancy is a time to develop habits of respecting your body, regardless of your previous schedules or work commitments. Even the most energetic women slow down in the early months of pregnancy. I can remember feeling ready for bed by seven and sleeping 10 or 12 hours at a stretch.

Short naps during the day can be a big help. If you have other small children, bundle everyone (yourself included) into a big bed in mid-afternoon for a story and a snooze. Children appreciate the chance for extra cuddling time with Mom and you get to really relax a bit before moving on to dinner preparation. Even a three-year-old child can learn to give you the kind of back rub you like—and will be eager to do it if you return the favor!

Short naps are a lifesaver when you have other children and work, too.

Meeting your needs for rest and sleep makes you more effective at the jobs you *have* to do and gives you a good reason for postponing or canceling things you prefer not to do. You deserve all the rest you can get, so be legitimately selfish with your time. Turn down that additional committee assignment for your civic group or a new work schedule that is incompatible with the needs of your pregnancy. If you are obligated to travel, entertain, redecorate, move, or assume care of an ailing friend or relative, try to plan it for the middle of pregnancy when you will probably feel more enterprising.

I found it much easier to say no during pregnancy.

Mid-Pregnancy

By the end of the third month of pregnancy, your baby is fully 3½ inches long and weighs an ounce. Months four through six see rapid growth and increasing refinement of system function. Your baby will achieve a length of 10 to 12 inches and a weight of 1½ to 2 pounds. His/her skeleton begins to harden into bone, tooth buds are formed in the gums, and the eyes are structurally complete and open for the first time. A thick layer of vernix (a cold cream-like substance) coats the baby's skin and protects it from constant exposure to its saline surroundings; fingernails and toenails appear; and the baby moves freely and vigorously, alternating periods of activity with periods of quiet. The baby's heartbeat can usually be picked up with the aid of a stethoscope from the fourth month on. It registers 120 to 160 beats a minute—about twice your rate. Your baby's growth spurt is reflected in the size of your uterus: By the fifth month, you can feel the fundus at the level of your navel.

All this growth, of course, depends on the continually expanding placenta which, in turn, requires an ever-increasing supply of blood to function optimally. As discussed in chapter 2, eating a balanced diet with enough protein, calories, and salt for pregnancy insures that the extra blood will be available. Providing the liver with the nutrients it needs keeps the essential fluid in your bloodstream. By five months gestation, the healthy placenta covers over 50 percent of the surface of the uterine wall. The marked increase in blood volume and demand on liver function to service the placenta are two changes you cannot detect by looking, yet they are crucial to the outcome of your pregnancy. Failure of the blood volume to expand results in damage to organs throughout the body, a malfunctioning placenta, intrauterine growth retardation for the baby, and metabolic toxemia for the mother. Preventing reduced blood volume (hypovolemia) prevents these conditions, regardless of the mother's age or previous obstetrical history.

During the second half of pregnancy, your breasts begin the phase of milk production. Under the influence of the hormone prolactin, the alveoli secrete colostrum, the thick, golden fluid especially adapted to the needs of the newborn. During pregnancy, prolactin is manufactured by the placenta. After birth, the suckling of the baby stimulates nerve endings in your nipple which triggers the release of prolactin and, subsequently, production of milk. The more often you put your baby to breast, the more milk you will have—a classic example of supply responding to demand. Other factors enter into breastfeeding as a mothering style, of course, but it is reassuring to know that your body is capable of nourishing your baby through such a simple and pleasurable mechanism.

Basic Breast Preparation

Your new baby will probably want to be at the breast more or less continuously for the first two or three days. Whether your nipples need advance conditioning for this workout depends on your skin type and the degree to which your nipples project when stimulated. Generally, the fairer your complexion, the more likely you are to develop sore nipples in the early days of nursing. A basic routine of breast preparation takes only a few minutes each day in the last half of pregnancy:

- At home, turn down the flaps of your nursing bras; so air circulates to the nipples, and they become somewhat desensitized by rubbing against the fabric of your blouse or sweater.
- Avoid the use of soap on your nipples. During pregnancy, they secrete their own protective film which keeps them supple and elastic. Plain water is all you need to cleanse them.
- After bathing, find a sunny spot, and expose your breasts to sunlight for a few minutes.
- Dab 100 percent plain lanolin on the areola and work it in by supporting the breast with one hand and repeatedly pulling the nipple outward with the other hand until the lanolin is absorbed. Plain lanolin can be purchased in small tubes from your pharmacy—a little goes a long way. Be wary of using anything else on your breasts and *never* use a preparation containing alcohol. If you do, you run the risk of drying out the nipples, leading to painful cracks and a higher risk of breast infection.
- Encourage your man to help in preparing for breastfeeding by massaging your breasts and stimulating them orally during lovemaking. Many women find that they can be aroused to orgasm during pregnancy by breast stimulation alone. It may be that the nerve

I am convinced that it's important to prepare your breasts before birth. I didn't and was in lots of pain and discomfort for four to five weeks after birth during nursing.

No one talks of the early physical discomforts of nursing —the pain—the feeling of not wanting to put the baby on the breast because of the pain, but wanting to because you know it will get better. The bond is so special. I had terrible pain for four to five weeks, especially on one side, so I finally used a sunlamp at night for weeks. Everything I read said the discomfort was minimal, but most women I spoke with agreed that they had pain. It would be easier to deal with the pain if one knew about the discomfort ahead of time.

I never had sore nipples. After each nursing, I applied lanolin and massaged it into the areola and nipple. This seemed to keep my skin elastic even when the baby wanted to suck for long periods of time and every hour or so.

endings in the nipple are more sensitive during pregnancy and lactation. At any rate, it is one more very persuasive reason for choosing to breast-feed.

Check the type of nipple you have by squeezing the areola between thumb and forefinger, then releasing it. Most nipples project after this test; some draw back and have to be coaxed outward by applying pressure on the surrounding breast tissue, then moving fingers back and forth to stretch the connective tissue at the base of the nipple. The truly inverted nipple is one which looks retracted all the time. The Woolwich breast shield may be purchased through your local La Leche League group and used from mid-pregnancy until birth to gently exert pressure on the nipple, pushing it through a center opening. Even the most resistant cases respond to the Woolwich shield if it is used faithfully.

Late Pregnancy

During the last six weeks of pregnancy, your baby gains an ounce a day, laying down a protective layer of fat that aids in regulating his/her body temperature after birth. But the most amazing development during the last two months is the staggeringly complex process of brain maturation. It is at this time that the higher functions of the brain begin to appear. Centers for voluntary muscular movement, coordination, sensory experience, memory, imagination, and intelligence are formed as the ten billion cells which comprise the brain interconnect. British and American research has conclusively shown that proper diet during these last few weeks of pregnancy is essential for optimum development of the brain and central nervous system. Undernutrition during the last few weeks can result in a baby who is severely mentally retarded, even though not of low birth weight (less than 5½ pounds). For these reasons, maintaining an adequate diet is of supreme importance every day until you go into labor.

Other profound adjustments take place in preparation for your baby's birth day:

Your joints relax in response to the huge amounts of hormones the placenta manufactures, allowing more give in the pelvic area through which your baby must pass en route to the outside world.

Your love partner may taste the sweetness of colostrum while licking your breasts.

Your cervix starts to soften markedly so that it can be dilated by the contractions of labor.

You feel more pressure on your bladder as your seven-to ten-pound baby descends further into the pelvis.

This pregnancy was a sheer joy. I felt exuberant at all times, radiant, and literally bursting with energy. My workload was a heavy one: I awoke each morning, quite early—5:30 a.m.—did my morning exercise routine, showered, dressed, ate breakfast, got my son off to school, straightened the house briefly, and then drove 45 minutes to my school. In addition to being a full-time wife, mother, and housekeeper, I was also a commuting three-quarter-time student in an interdisciplinary premed and nutrition program. On top of all that, I was also deeply involved in the local school district lunch program and in our food cooperative. When spring rolled around, I even found enough energy to plant our annual vegetable garden. So when I say I felt energetic, I truly mean it!

You are more aware at times of your uterus becoming very hard—often when you roll from side to side during the night or change position from sitting to standing. These tightenings are Braxton-Hicks contractions which "tune-up" the uterus for the more vigorous events of true labor.

Your face may be rounded out, your fingers swollen so you can't remove your rings, and your feet puffy so that the only comfortable shoes are flat sandals. All of this is perfectly normal in any well-fed mother, due to the placental hormones causing you to retain fluid so you do not become dehydrated during labor. You also have about 50 percent more blood circulating through your body, another safeguard for birth when some blood loss is unavoidable.

During the last few weeks, you will probably welcome opportunities to nap or rest, much as you did in the first trimester. Your body is heavier, you move more slowly, your nighttime sleep is interrupted by the baby's movements and your own needs to urinate or just to think about the marvels occurring within you. Pay attention to the feelings you have, and get enough rest.

There is no worse enemy during labor than fatigue. The process of giving birth can take 24 hours or more in some mothers, depending on the size and position of the baby, the size and shape of your pelvis, and the strength and coordination of your contractions. Realize that *your* labor might last that long, and be realistic about the rest you need.

Labor and Birth

Giving birth is the female's opportunity to experience her body at its most elemental and powerful. Just as passionate lovemaking brings about overwhelming, driving waves of physical sensation, intense emotion, and profound release and satisfaction afterward, bringing forth a child follows much the same course. When you consider that this process occurs independently of the will of the mother, at its own speed and rhythm, and on its own terms, suggestions for labor preparation can be summarized in one sentence: *Learn how to cooperate with it!*

The basic unit of labor is the uterine contraction. During each contraction the uterine ligaments pull up on themselves, gradually drawing the cervix apart and taking it up into the uterine wall itself. At the same time, pressure from the top of the uterus, the fundus, presses the baby farther down into the pelvic basin, speeding the opening up of the cervix and hastening the time for actually pushing the baby out.

Once the cervix has been fully dilated, the uterus, aided by the bearing-down efforts of the abdominal muscles, moves the baby through the vagina and out of the mother's body. The force of the contractions propels the baby through the birth canal so that even the biggest proportions (usually head and shoulders) assume the smallest diameters for passing through the arches of the bony pelvis. This adjustment is assisted by the molding of the baby's head to the mother's birth canal, made possible because the bones of the baby's skull are still very pliable at birth.

The placenta gradually separates from the uterine wall after the baby is out. It is expelled with one final contraction as the last step in the birth process.

Uterus at Work! Keep the Rest of Your Body Out of the Way!

By the time your labor is ready to begin, the uterus is the largest muscle in your body. When it contracts, especially in the urgent phase of transition, it is the primary physical event taking place in your body. To pretend that it isn't happening or to try to do something else while it is happening is to doom yourself to an unnecessarily difficult and tiring labor experience. The most intelligent approach to labor is to keep the rest of your body out of the way of the working uterus. This means conserving energy during the long first stage of cervical dilation so that you have enough strength left to push your baby out during the expulsive stage.

The key to conservation of energy during labor and *allowing your body to have the baby* is training in progressive relaxation. Ideally, you and your partner should begin this training midway through your pregnancy so that you are experts by the time your baby is due. It is helpful, but not absolutely necessary, to work with an experienced instructor as you master the simple techniques of progressive relaxation that constitute part of Cooperative Childbirth.

Cooperative Childbirth means that the mother learns to cooperate with her body, and everyone else learns to cooperate with the mother. These concepts form the foundation of the childbirth education program offered by the Childbirth Education Association of Metropolitan New York and the Cooperative Childbirth Network. Classes offered by teachers affiliated with the American Academy of Husband-Coached Childbirth (The Bradley Method) also stress progressive relaxation.

Progressive Relaxation

The principles of progressive relaxation have been known since 1920 when Dr. Edmund Jacobson of Harvard

During my labor, there were occasions when I suddenly felt a need to squat, or to breathe deeply, or to pace around, or to kneel on the floor. I could sense inner changes, and I could feel the rhythm of birth with its increasing crescendo inside my whole being. No attendant was there to say how much I had dilated, or if I had begun transition—and what did that matter anyway? I relied on my own ability to listen to my body, to pay close heed to its changes, and to respond to them as only I knew how.

Relaxation does it all! I reached the hospital in transition, but because I could relax with each contraction, I thought I was in early labor or false labor. With my first labor the pain was unbearable, and I demanded drugs. This time, I couldn't believe I was already in transition—it wasn't painful enough!

began publishing articles in medical journals on the use of relaxation training to combat nervous tension. His 1934 classic, *You Must Relax* (New York: McGraw-Hill Book Co.), now in its fifth edition (1976), discussed practical methods for reducing tension in everyday life and his *How to Relax and Have Your Baby* (New York: McGraw-Hill Book Co.) appeared in 1959.

The thrust of progressive relaxation is to train an individual to recognize tension in various muscle groups throughout the body and to be able to release it at will. The goal during childbirth is to do *no work* with muscles not directly involved in the process of giving birth and to maximize the comfort of the mother throughout labor and birth.

Two physicians who were pioneers in the field of natural childbirth, Grantly Dick-Read in the 1930s and Robert A. Bradley since the 1940s, both reached the above conclusions about childbirth education after being distressed by the prevailing mode of obstetrical practice—heavy on medication and light on preparation for labor. Their respective books, *Childbirth Without Fear* (New York: Harper & Row) and *Husband-Coached Childbirth* (New York: Harper & Row), have provided many women with guidelines for natural childbirth with or without support from their physicians. Though some of the attitudes and language in these books seem dated, the essence of the method remains valid for any woman seeking the least-stressful way of having a baby. These considerations rank high on the list of concerns for older mothers who may have been told by physicians that they should anticipate a great deal of trouble in giving birth.

Women with previous disappointing birth experiences also need special attention during the current pregnancy to overcome the feeling that their bodies don't work well during labor and can't be trusted. Training in progressive relaxation helps the mother become better acquainted with her body during pregnancy and increases her feelings of confidence about the approaching labor.

Relaxation Practice

The objective of relaxation practice is to develop skills of muscular release that can be employed during labor. Like any other sort of physical skill, progressive relaxation requires practice in order to be perfected. The ability to release muscle groups consciously throughout the body while uterine contractions increase in intensity is not a function of just knowing, intellectually, what has to be done. It is *doing* it!

In the case of the woman in labor, it means the ability to do it whenever and wherever the labor takes place, no matter who else is there. Despite our best-laid plans, labor does not always occur under the best circumstances, so it is in your best interest to practice for any and all eventualities.

Learning to cooperate with your body can be a challenging task. Though the techniques may seem transparently clear to the mind, they may present themselves in a different way to your body. When you choose to use progressive relaxation as the fundamental tool for managing your labor experience, you are aiming to achieve physical repose and keep mentally alert *simultaneously,* while your body is undergoing physiologic stress (uterine contractions).

Since your training is designed to make you aware of what true relaxation feels like in your own body, your goal during labor is to duplicate the same feelings of release that you attained during practice.

Having a labor partner who has gone though training with you and is an expert in recognizing your characteristic responses to physical stress is a decided advantage. The partner can keep a careful eye on your responses to the contractions and maintain an objectivity about the process that will be impossible for you as your body becomes caught up in its powerful work. Progressive relaxation is a specific plan implemented for labor. It is not transcendental meditation, yoga, positive thinking, or plain old loafing!

Get to Know the Feeling of True Release

The first step in relaxation training is to become aware of what your body feels like when it is truly released. Spending a few minutes before bedtime analyzing how you go to sleep will raise your awareness of what *your* comfort rituals are. Each of us finds positions for sleep that are most comfortable. The covers must be fixed a certain way, the room darkened, our loved ones close by, a favorite record playing—all examples of the aids to relaxation that can easily be used during labor.

Most pregnant women find lying on their sides or propped at a 45-degree angle more comfortable than lying on the back or stomach. To facilitate comfort even more, the mother needs to make a "nest" for herself with pillows. The reason: One cardinal rule for achieving relaxation anywhere is that *every joint be bent and every joint be supported.* The limbs, back, and neck should be doing *no work.* The eyes close to eliminate distractions. Breathing slows and becomes deeper as relaxation extends throughout the body. Your partner can check your relaxation by

Relaxation worked well for me. I got through every part of early labor—except for pushing—at home. My contractions were irregular, so we spent the night waiting for them to become regular. We watched TV and I talked on the phone while I lay in bed. I walked around from room to room, too. The contractions were bearable at all times. I minded them least when standing with my head against my husband's shoulder while he stroked my back. This, purists will say, isn't complete relaxation—which kind of proves it's how you're feeling mentally that counts the most. Being with my husband and being at home made the difference.

When I got to the hospital I was 9½ centimeters dilated. But the labor seemed to have stopped. I had no urge to push. They broke the bag of waters, but still my contractions wouldn't come unless I provoked them by hunching over. Finally, after three hours of pushing, the baby was born.

She cried once as she was born. She was given to me immediately and sucked right away. Her eyes were wide, looking into mine.

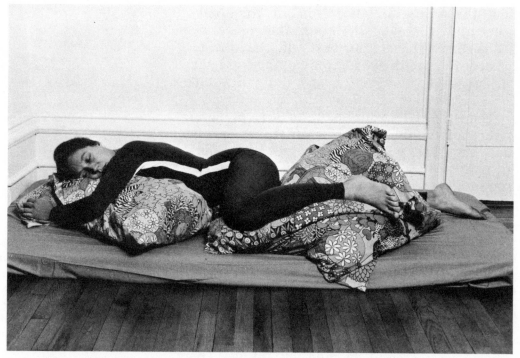

Nest of pillows aids relaxation.

gently lifting hands or feet and letting them flop back onto the bed or pillows supporting you. Eventually, you should have the feeling that the bed is doing the work and your body is completely at rest. This is the state you aim to duplicate in labor. Remember that the objective is to save energy during the first stage of labor by not interfering with the action of the uterus.

Once you have the basic sense of relaxation in your own body, you can help your partner detect variations with these additional techniques.

I had so much energy left that Rachel was out in three good pushes.

- Tense and release specific body parts starting at the forehead, moving downward through cheeks, jaw, tongue, neck, shoulders, arms, fingers, back, buttocks, thighs, calves, and feet.

  Have your partner place a hand on the part being tensed, and keep it there until you release it. This gives the partner a chance to actually feel the difference between a tense muscle and a released one. This is a fundamental skill for labor when the partner has to detect tension of which you may not even be aware.

A partner is essential. My husband kept bringing me back to relaxation whenever I began to tighten up.

- Teach your partner how to give you a back rub. The aim is to increase your comfort; so the pressure, type of

RELAXATION PRACTICE

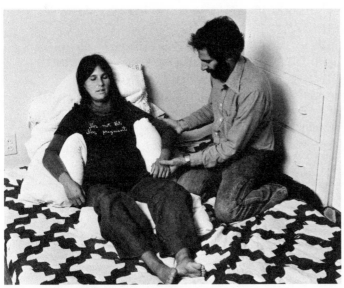

1—In 45-degree position:
   every joint bent, every joint supported
   . . . head, arms, and knees.

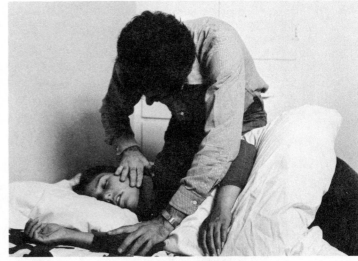

2—In side position:
   release facial muscles.

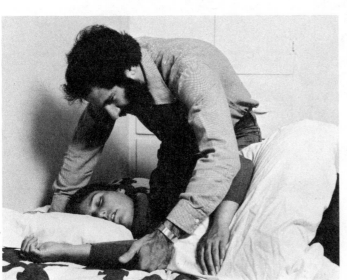

3—Support upper arm with pillow,
   release arms and hands.

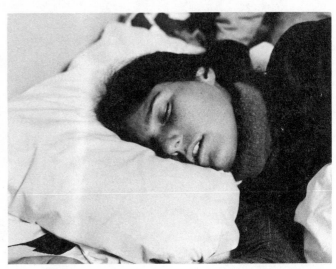

4—Open mouth. . .
   body at rest.

stroking, and pace is up to you. What you like now may not feel good in labor, so remind your partner that you may need a different kind of touching in labor. Use a pillow tucked in at the lower back to enable you to really let those large back muscles go, and save a lot of unnecessary energy expenditure.

- Simulate the painful stress of contractions by having your partner pinch you with varying degrees of strength (work up to full-grip strength gradually as your ability to release during stress improves) on various parts of your body. These pinches do not feel anything like a real contraction, but they are good practice. It gives your partner a chance to become familiar with your charac-

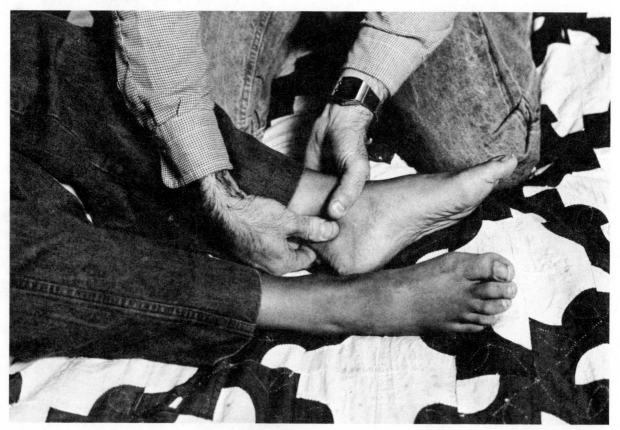

SIMULATED CONTRACTION
Partner pinches on vulnerable spot. Mother practices release while experiencing pain.

Strength of Uterine Contractions

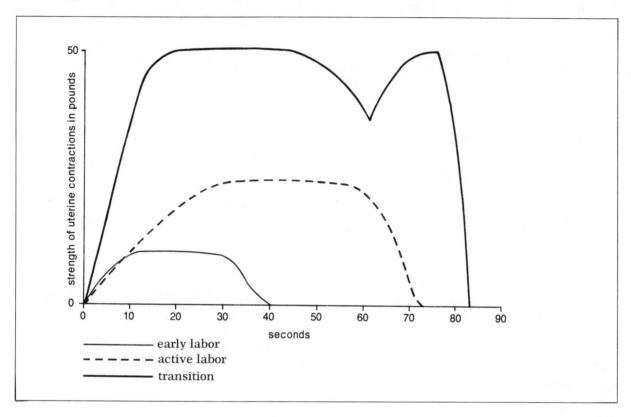

teristic response to pain and with ways he can soothe whatever muscle group you are tensing.

The pinch of a simulated contraction should follow the pattern of a classic contraction at first. Later in your preparation, you can add contractions with double and triple peaks and those which start off at the peak—all of which are likely during the most intense phase of labor, just before the cervix is fully dilated.

As far as actual labor goes, the only important contraction is the one you're having. Deal with each one as it presents itself, then let it go. Never predict the future of your labor. This contraction may be the last. Never think back to contractions you have already dealt with. They will never return. Stay in the present time and focus your attention on what you can do to release tension *now*. One of the absolute tip-offs that you are completely relaxed is when you find yourself drooling on the pillow.

Family-Centered Childbirth and Parenting of Fulton, New York, has developed a Labor Readiness Scale to help parents evaluate their labor practice sessions.

My ability to relax and let my whole body sag as each contraction began and Al's (my husband) expert back massage at the site to which I directed him, led to a relatively easy, relaxed, first delivery. I had back labor, too, which should have made my labor more difficult. We owe the ease of the labor to all we learned with a course on the Bradley Method of Husband-Coached Childbirth: how to work as a team and how to relax.

Labor Readiness Scale

Note: You and your partner should answer questions separately, compare your answers, and see where you can improve. Instructions for scoring and interpreting your answers follow.

SECTION I. READINESS FOR LABOR

1. How often do you practice coaching and relaxation together each week?
   a. once
   b. twice
   c. three times
   d. four times
   e. five or more times

2. How well do you feel you and your partner relax as a team?
   a. very well
   b. well
   c. fairly well
   d. okay
   e. poorly

3. When practicing relaxation together, how often do you feel you or your partner has trouble with giggling or joking?
   a. almost every time
   b. about half the time
   c. about a quarter of the time
   d. rarely
   e. never

4. During coaching and relaxation practice, do you feel that your partner is overly critical?
   a. never
   b. rarely
   c. occasionally
   d. frequently
   e. always

5. What is the average length of the times you practice coaching and relaxation (think in terms of the last three weeks)?
   a. 30 minutes
   b. 20 minutes
   c. 15 minutes
   d. 10 minutes
   e. 5 minutes

6. Do you practice coaching and relaxation when you feel upset or distracted?
   a. always
   b. frequently
   c. occasionally
   d. rarely
   e. never

7. When practicing together, how often do you criticize your partner's efforts?
   a. never
   b. rarely
   c. occasionally
   d. frequently
   e. every time

8. When practicing relaxation and coaching, do you find that you (the mother) drool?
   a. always
   b. often
   c. occasionally
   d. rarely
   e. never

9. When practicing together, which relaxation techniques do you use?
   a. coaching breathing with counting
   b. imagining a relaxing scene
   c. alternately tensing and relaxing parts of the body
   d. love talk
   e. touching or talking while relaxing various parts of the body
   f. rubbing and caressing

10. Who takes the lead in seeing that relaxation and coaching are practiced?
    a. always you
    b. always your partner
    c. mostly you
    d. mostly your partner
    e. equally responsible

11. How do you rate your confidence that you can do your part in labor and delivery?
    a. completely confident
    b. very confident
    c. confident
    d. unsure of yourself
    e. very unsure of yourself

12. How do you rate your partner's confidence that he or she can do his or her part?
    a. completely confident
    b. very confident
    c. confident
    d. unsure
    e. very unsure

13. Do you feel you have a good knowledge of what to expect in labor?
    a. poor knowledge
    b. so-so knowledge
    c. good knowledge
    d. very good knowledge
    e. excellent knowledge

14. Do you feel your partner has a good knowledge of what to expect in labor?
    a. excellent knowledge
    b. very good knowledge
    c. good knowledge
    d. so-so knowledge
    e. poor knowledge

15. Do you expect to enjoy your birth experience?
    a. not at all
    b. very little
    c. some
    d. quite a bit
    e. immensely

16. Do you feel your partner expects to enjoy his or her birth experience?
    a. not at all
    b. very little
    c. some
    d. quite a bit
    e. immensely

17. Do you and your partner have a hard time getting into coaching and relaxation?
    a. a very hard time
    b. hard
    c. not hard
    d. fairly easy
    e. easy

18. When you and your partner practice relaxation and coaching, do you find it boring?
    a. very often
    b. often
    c. sometimes
    d. seldom
    e. rarely

19. Do you feel your partner worries that he or she can't do natural childbirth?
    a. almost never
    b. rarely
    c. sometimes
    d. frequently

20. How often do you worry that you can't do natural childbirth?
    a. frequently
    b. sometimes
    c. rarely
    d. almost never

21. When practicing relaxation, do you or your partner have difficulty staying in the present and concentrating on relaxation?
    a. always
    b. usually
    c. sometimes
    d. rarely
    e. never

22. When practicing relaxation, do you or your partner keep thinking of things you should be doing, or tasks (other than relaxation) you have to do later?
    a. always
    b. usually
    c. sometimes
    d. rarely
    e. never

23. When practicing relaxation and coaching, do you find yourselves quarreling?
    a. never
    b. rarely
    c. sometimes
    d. often
    e. every time

SECTION II. PERFORMANCE AS A TEAM DURING PREGNANCY

1. Are you and your partner in complete agreement about what you want your birth experience to include?   Yes/No

2. Have you and your partner visited the doctor together?   Yes/No

3. Have you worked out a completely satisfactory arrangement with your doctor or midwife regarding what should and should not happen during your birth experience?   Yes/No

4. Have you attended all the classes together?   Yes/No

5. Have both of you done the reading?   Yes/No

6. Do you occasionally quiz each other on aspects of labor and delivery out of class?   Yes/No

7. As a couple, have you successfully fended off fears and doubts spread by tellers of old wives' tales?   Yes/No

8. Do you feel completely assured that you and your partner have made adequate plans and preparations for taking it easy during the first two weeks after your baby is born?   Yes/No

9. Is the female member of your team doing all the exercises every day?   Yes/No

10. Have you both faced the fact that staying in good physical and emotional shape as your due date nears and then passes requires that you limit your social and business commitments?   Yes/No

11. Have you changed your diet to include enough protein, calories, salt, vitamins, and minerals?   Yes/No

12. Have you made the financial arrangements for your baby's birth in advance?   Yes/No

13. Have you asked all the questions you have had, either in class or at your appointments with your doctor?   Yes/No

SCORING INSTRUCTIONS

Section I.

1. a: 1 b: 2 c: 3 d: 4 e: 5	5. a: 5 b: 4 c: 3 d: 2 e: 1	9. a thru f, score 1 each up to a total of 5 points.	13. a: 1 b: 2 c: 3 d: 4 e: 5	17. a: 1 b: 2 c: 3 d: 4 e: 5	21. a: 1 b: 2 c: 3 d: 4 e: 5
2. a: 5 b: 4 c: 3 d: 2 e: 1	6. a: 1 b: 2 c: 3 d: 4 e: 5	10. a: 1 b: 1 c: 2 d: 2 e: 4	14. a: 5 b: 4 c: 3 d: 2 e: 1	18. a: 1 b: 2 c: 3 d: 4 e: 5	22. a: 1 b: 2 c: 3 d: 4 e: 5
3. a: 1 b: 2 c: 3 d: 4 e: 5	7. a: 1 b: 2 c: 3 d: 4 e: 5	11. a: 5 b: 4 c: 3 d: 2 e. 1	15. a: 1 b: 2 c: 3 d: 4 e: 5	19. a: 4 b: 3 c: 2 d: 1	23. a: 5 b: 4 c: 3 d: 2 e: 1
4. a: 5 b: 4 c: 3 d: 2 e: 1	8. a: 5 b: 4 c: 3 d: 2 e: 1	12. a: 5 b: 4 c: 3 d: 2 e: 1	16. a: 1 b: 2 c: 3 d: 4 e: 5	20. a: 1 b: 2 c: 3 d: 4	24. a: 5 b: 4 c: 3 d: 2 e: 1

Section II.

Score 1 point for each yes answer, 0 for each no answer.

WHAT THESE SCORES MEAN

Section I.   95 and up—good, keep it up. 81 to 94—poor, needs lots of work. 80 and below—desperate, requires *special help*.

Section II.   10 to 13—good. 8 to 9—poor, it's time to face facts and get things straightened out. 7 and below—desperate. *Special help* needed.

EXPLANATION OF SCORE INTERPRETATION

The scores for sections I and II measure different things and should not be combined for an average score. If your scores for either section are low, review the questions and answers for that section to determine where you are weak, then *act* to strengthen yourselves in that area. Also, if one person has high scores but the other member of your team has a low score, it is the *low score* that counts. A team is only as strong as its weakest member. Don't lay blame or make excuses; just do something about it.

This Scale is for your use, not your instructor's. It is intended to warn you of areas that need work and to motivate you to do that work. The responsibility is yours. Sometimes, however, couples need outside help in working to improve their handling of childbirth preparation. If your scores fell in the desperate category, you ought to consider seeking such help from your instructors, a marriage counselor, or some other individual who can help you clarify your goals, develop a better working relationship, and improve your practicing techniques.

Birth Preferences

It is possible to accomplish the kind of birth that is most healthful for you and your baby in almost any institutional setting if you know one simple fact: *You have the right to refuse any treatment, medication, procedure, or personnel simply by informing the person offering it to you that you do not give your consent.*

Most of us have been led to believe that we have to accept whatever the hospital policies are regarding birth practices. In effect, we sign a paper that theoretically gives the hospital absolute rights over our person while we are using the hospital facilities. In actuality, those forms mean little, and no nurse or other hospital employee will try to force you to accept a procedure when you make it clear that you know it is within your rights to refuse it.

It is not easy to say no when you are being intimidated with insinuations that unless you accept the medication or procedure, you are jeopardizing the welfare of your baby or yourself. However, when you have a clear understanding of the dynamics of normal birth and the assurance that you have taken all the possible precautions against a poor outcome during your pregnancy, the problems associated with giving birth in an American hospital can be surmounted.

Have a Labor Partner with You

Of course, it is much easier when you have a labor partner who has attended childbirth education classes with you and is ready to "run interference" with the hospital staff for you. Under ideal circumstances, this person is your baby's father, but anyone you feel comfortable with (sister, mother, friend) can assist you in labor.

Even when both parents have attended classes, they often like to have a third person accompany them to the hospital so they can concentrate on giving birth while their advocate runs for ice chips, extra pillows, makes phone calls, and advises nurses when the mother wishes to consult with them.

In the early part of this century, when hospital birth was just becoming established for all women, it was common for women who could afford it to hire a private duty nurse to be their companion during labor and birth. This service is now being performed in some parts of the country by women trained specifically as labor attendants. They appreciate that labor and birth are also exceptional emotional experiences for fathers, so their concern today is for the

We used the opportunity to learn as much as we could about pregnancy and labor. I took an active role with my physicians and knew what I expected from them. The results were rewarding: My labor experience and the delivery of our son will always be cherished by my husband and me as among the most intimate, intensely beautiful experiences of our lives. We look forward to our next time with eager anticipation.

After a true natural birth, the nurse began to inject me with Pitocin. My husband jumped up and asked her to take the needle away. The nurse looked at the doctor and he said "OK, but if you start to hemorrhage you'll need it." From then on I was the patient who refused her Pitocin. And I didn't hemorrhage . . . nursing took care of my uterus.

couple—assisting both parents in attaining the hospital birth they desire.

An outline of birth preferences, discussed in detail with your doctor or midwife during a course of several prenatal visits well in advance of the birth, is often used by parents. When both parents are able to discuss their birth preferences with the medical attendant, and they provide a written list of their preferences to be initialed by the doctor and attached to their prenatal chart, they are much more likely to have their births handled as they wish.

Distinguishing your preferences from those of the many other women using the physician or midwife you have chosen may take persistence. Obstetrical offices are usually full, waits are often long, and you may feel uneasy requesting more time for conversation than seems routine. However, unless you are specific about your preferences, you are likely to be treated in a routine manner when you arrive at the hospital in labor.

Many of the routine practices, such as removal of the pubic hair, administration of an enema, artificial rupture of membranes, confinement to bed, starting of intravenous fluids, sedation, and attachment to a fetal monitor are being vigorously challenged by consumer and professional groups. Many of these practices were originally intended for application in a select number of high-risk cases and are now being touted as preventive measures for all laboring women. Some of these practices, while traditional in American obstetrics, are now known to be causative of complications during labor and more likely to result in infections for mother and baby. In general, the Cooperative Childbirth Preferences outline which follows favors the most conservative medical/obstetrical practice whenever possible.

We visited the hospital where I was to give birth and came away with lots of negative feelings. However, our doctor was affiliated with this hospital, and we didn't want to change doctors. We put everything we expected from the hospital in writing, and our doctor signed the statement. We had a good birth because we did that. When any questions came up about drugs, anesthetics, my husband's presence, my nursing the baby and such, we just referred the hospital's personnel to our statement signed by the doctor.

---

*I saw a doctor in a clinic at the hospital I would be using for birth. My other children were born there, too, and I knew that they did not permit fathers in the labor room—in fact, all the women in labor were kept in one big room with rows of beds. Everyone was moaning and crying and screaming through the whole time. I had accepted drugs with the other babies because it was too painful and saddening to be left there all alone for hours with no way of defending yourself. With the first one, we had gone to a series of very fashion-*able Lamaze childbirth classes in a private Manhattan studio, and we had faithfully practiced the breathing—but the instructor never told us *the hospital didn't allow fathers in the labor or delivery rooms,* and we didn't know enough at the time to ask about it in advance. So, I was terribly upset when it didn't work out the way we had planned.

Of course, the doctor in the clinic never even knew my name and could just barely remember that I was the one who wanted to have her husband with her. This hospital services many Spanish-speaking women, and no attempt is made to offer childbirth preparation to them as part of their prenatal care so it's no wonder the medicated birth is still the rule. I gave the doctor a list of birth preferences from the Bradley class which he said he would attach to my chart. He never did this, as we found out later. He also kept saying he was trying to get my husband a permission note from the hospital administrator. I don't think he was doing that, either.

Cooperative Childbirth Preferences*

Part I: Labor

Preference	Rationale
1. Every mother is entitled to the continuous companionship of at least one person of her choice throughout labor, birth, and the early postpartum hours.	1. A trained labor partner is a source of unparalleled support, both psychological and physical, for the laboring woman.
2. Partner(s) should remain with mother during all admission procedures, especially if she is in advanced labor.	2. Separation from her support person can trigger anxiety and interfere with mother's ability to relax during contractions.
3. Encourage ambulation as desired by the mother.	3. Uterine contractions are most efficient when mother is in an upright position and free to move about between contractions.
4. Refrain from routine use of IV fluids.	4. Well-nourished mothers have expanded plasma volume and stored fluid as prophylaxes against dehydration and shock. A mother who gives birth spontaneously, without analgesia or anesthesia, and breast-feeds her baby at birth rarely hemorrhages. IV interferes with relaxation.
5. Encourage mother to adapt her position during labor to facilitate comfort. Aim to cooperate with the working uterus by doing as little work as possible with other muscle groups.	5. Standing, sitting, hands-and-knees, or lying on one's side may be appropriate in individual cases. Laboring on the back reduces circulation to legs, placenta, and baby; reduces efficiency of contractions; and is more painful for mother.
6. Provide ice chips, liquids, and extra pillows as requested by mother.	6. Mouth may become dry from loose-jaw breathing. Pillows aid in relaxation: EVERY JOINT BENT, EVERY JOINT SUPPORTED is the key to muscle release.

*A reprint may be ordered for 25¢ from: Cooperative Childbirth Network, 14 Truesdale Drive, Croton-on-Hudson, NY 10520. Send a stamped, self-addressed envelope with request. Bulk-order information also available.

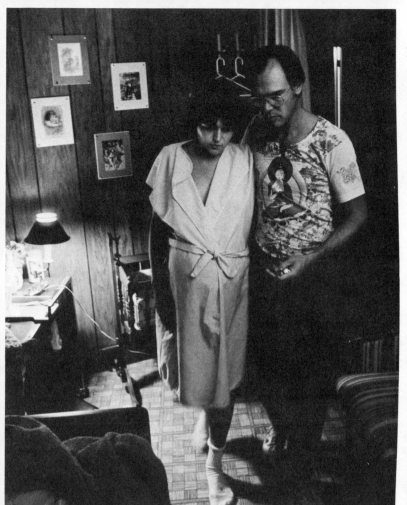

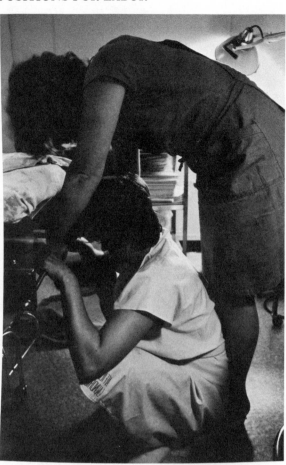

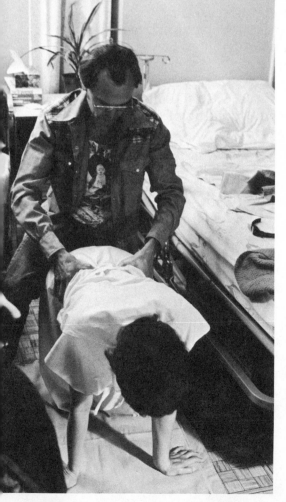

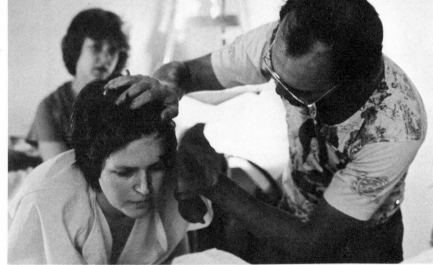

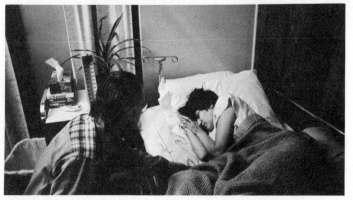

Adapt labor positions to facilitate mother's comfort.

Preference	Rationale
7. Breathing responds to mother's need for oxygen and reflects her level of relaxation.	7. Rote repetition of unphysiologic breathing patterns wastes energy. PROGRESSIVE RELAXATION is the fundamental skill for labor. Extended periods of panting can cause hyperventilation. Performance of any unnecessary activities interferes with relaxation.
8. Partner(s) should be present during examinations or other procedures that become necessary.	8. See rationale number 2.
9. Provide clear information on the progress of labor to mother and partner(s). Refrain from predicting future events or the length of labor remaining. Encourage the mother to concentrate only on the contraction she is having at the present time.	9. The mother and labor partner(s) may wish to adjust their techniques based on information provided. Back rub, touch relaxation, verbal support, and adjusting bed are direct aids partner performs, as practiced extensively in class.
10. Assist in creating a calm, restful atmosphere in labor room.	10. Loud discussions, unnecessary interference during contractions, separating mother and partner, harsh lighting, and impersonal attitudes hinder relaxation and concentration.
11. Allow membranes to rupture spontaneously.	11. Forewaters provide a cushioning effect, equalizing pressure on the baby's head during contractions. Excessive molding of the head is caused by unequal pressure after amniotomy. Artificial rupture commits staff to delivery by schedule and increases the risk of infection to mother and baby.
12. Induction, augmentation, and stimulation of labor should be reserved for cases of medical necessity.	12. Known dangers of induction to mother and baby (prolapse of cord, prematurity, tetanic contractions) are compounded by the difficulty a mother may have in maintaining relaxation during accelerated labor with intense contractions.
13. Encourage the use of labor-delivery beds, either in labor room or wheeled into delivery room at appropriate time.	13. It is awkward and upsetting to the mother to be moved during period of transition/pushing. Adjustable beds can be adapted to the needs of

Preference	Rationale
	individual mothers for the most efficient birth position requiring the least amount of exertion.
14. Partner(s) should dress for the delivery room soon after admission to the labor unit and stay with the mother during transfer to the delivery room.	14. A mother should not be subjected to unnecessary stress during her most difficult time of labor. Her partner is trained to help her find the most comfortable pushing position and to give verbal support.

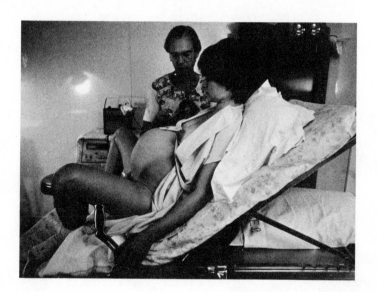

Part II: Birth

1. If using conventional delivery table, do not break.	1. Mother needs a place to rest her legs between contractions.
2. DO NOT RESTRAIN MOTHER'S ARMS OR LEGS. DO NOT PLACE IN LITHOTOMY POSITION.	2. Mother needs freedom to adjust her pushing efforts as directed by attendants. In the modified squatting position, propped at a 45-degree angle, the attendant's vision is unobstructed. Mother wishes to give birth, not be delivered.
3. Encourage mother to release breath during pushing contractions.	3. This allows the baby to emerge gently from the mother's body and reduces stress on the abdominal muscles (*diastasis recti*) and pelvic floor.
4. Wait until the height of a contraction late in the second	4. When legs are relaxed, not stretched wide with stirrups, and uterine

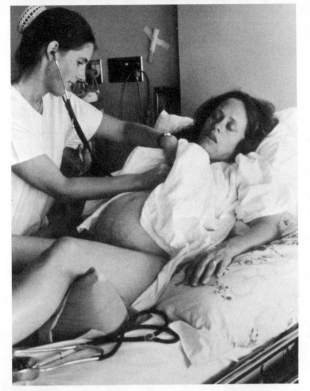

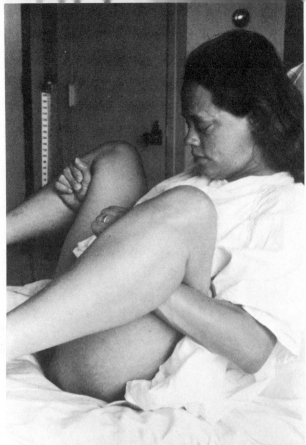

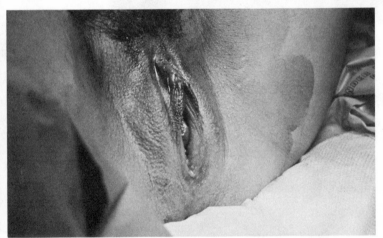

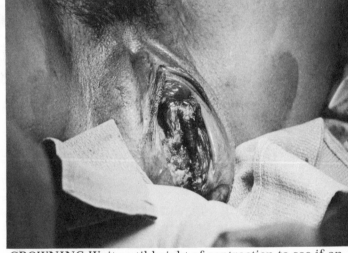

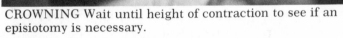

CROWNING Wait until height of contraction to see if an episiotomy is necessary.

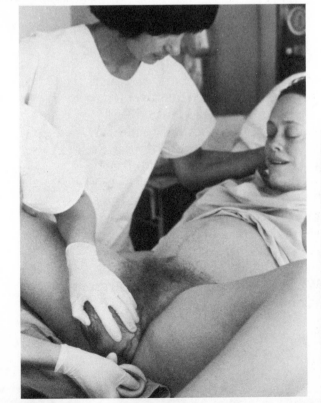

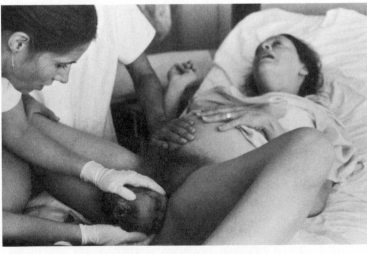

Preference	Rationale
stage to determine whether a pressure episiotomy is needed.	action alone is allowed to push the baby through the birth canal, trauma to the pelvic floor is minimized. There is more "give" in the muscles and tissues of a well-nourished mother, also. The pressure of the head against maternal tissues at the peak of a contraction provides numbness for incision, if needed.
5. Refrain from routine suctioning of newborn.	5. Babies born spontaneously to unmedicated mothers in physiologic position have most mucus expelled by the time of birth. The baby's chest is compressed by the vaginal walls during the second stage, so drainage is accomplished automatically. The baby continues to receive oxygen through the cord until it is severed.
6. Allow placental blood to transfuse through the cord before cutting.	6. Placental blood is part of the infant's circulation and is needed to perfuse the newly functioning bronchial tree. A smaller placenta results in a quicker third stage.
7. Give the infant directly to mother after birth, skin-to-skin. Cover both with receiving blanket to maintain warmth.	7. The period after birth is a highly sensitive time for mother and infant. Baby needs to be comforted by mother. Parents are aware of the appearance of a newborn. Mother is the best radiant heat source in room.
8. Encourage mother to breast-feed as soon as the baby seems calm.	8. Breast stimulation triggers release of oxytocin, causing rhythmic

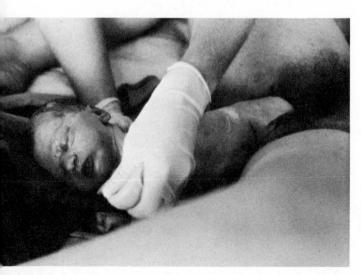

Moments after birth . . . mother and baby . . . skin-to-skin.

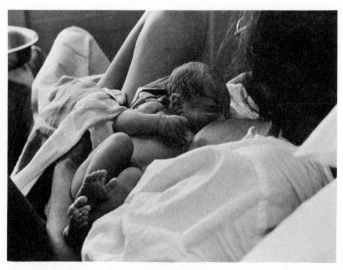

Preference	Rationale
Help mother introduce her nipple to the baby's mouth. The Apgar rating can be done while baby is at the breast. Nursing should continue until the placenta separates spontaneously from the uterine wall.	uterine contractions which gradually separate the placenta. PATIENCE is the key, not tugging on the cord, abdominal pressure, Ergotrate, or manual removal of placenta as may be necessary when the mother is anesthesized. Colostrum is vital for the newborn because of its antiinfective properties.
9. Repair episiotomy, if done, with a local anesthesia. Father has time to hold infant.	9. A local does not impede normal motor or eliminative functions. It is simple and quick to administer.
10. Serve orange juice or other fruit juice.	10. This restores blood sugar to normal levels without need for an IV.
11. Mother and baby should continue breast-feeding uninterrupted during early postpartum hours. Parents should accompany baby to the nursery for evaluation, then return to the labor suite or to postpartum floor with the baby.	11. Mother may walk as soon as she feels like it. This restores circulation to the pelvic area. Continuous nursing serves as a prophylaxis against hemorrhage. A mother is able and desirous of caring for her baby. Parents may wish to bathe infant.
12. Mother and baby should be discharged as soon as they desire if there is no medical contraindication. Six to 24 hours is the typical stay for normal birth.	12. This minimizes conflicts caused by leaving other children at home and reduces the chances of baby and mother getting postpartum infection (staph). The infant is not subjected to a feeding schedule. Mother can rest better at home when other household work is done by another.
13. If mother stays longer in the hospital, she should have access to her baby whenever she desires. Baby should be brought to mother when crying.	13. Baby needs to feed when hungry. Experienced breast-feeding counselor should be available to assist mother with breastfeeding if needed. This is especially true when birth has been difficult or Cesarean has been performed.
14. Visits by other family members should be possible at regular intervals. Healthy siblings should be encouraged.	14. Frequent visits maintain the family as a unit and allow the mother to concentrate on her new baby without worry about the welfare of her other children.

Beyond this basic outline of an uncomplicated birth, parents need to know their rights and responsibilities when medical intervention is being contemplated. The right of every mother to make an informed decision and give her informed consent to every treatment or medication has been carefully explained in "The Pregnant Patient's Bill of Rights," a publication of the Committee on Patient's Rights which follows.

The Pregnant Patient's Bill of Rights

American parents are becoming increasingly aware that well-intentioned health professionals do not always have scientific data to support common American obstetrical practices and that many of these practices are carried out primarily because they are part of medical and hospital tradition. In the last forty years, many artificial practices have been introduced which have changed childbirth from a physiological event to a very complicated medical procedure in which all kinds of drugs are used and procedures carried out, sometimes unnecessarily, and many of them are potentially damaging for the baby and even for the mother. A growing body of research makes it alarmingly clear that every aspect of traditional American hospital care during labor and delivery must now be questioned as to its possible effect on the future well-being of both the obstetric patient and her unborn child.

One in every 35 children born in the United States today will eventually be diagnosed as retarded; in 75 percent of these cases, there is no familial or genetic predisposing factor. One in every 10 to 17 children has been found to have some form of brain dysfunction or learning disability requiring special treatment. Such statistics are not confined to the lower socioeconomic group but cut across all segments of American society.

New concerns are being raised by childbearing women, because no one knows what degree of oxygen depletion, head compression, or traction by forceps the unborn or newborn infant can tolerate before that child sustains permanent brain damage or dysfunction. The recent findings regarding the cancer-related drug diethylstilbestrol have alerted the public to the fact that neither the approval of a drug by the U. S. Food and Drug Administration nor the fact that a drug is prescribed by a physician serves as a guarantee that a drug or medication is safe for the mother or her unborn child. In fact, the American Academy of Pediatrics' Committee on Drugs has recently stated that there is no drug, whether prescription or over-the-counter remedy, which has been proven safe for the unborn child.

The Pregnant Patient has the right to participate in decisions involving her well-being and that of her unborn child, unless there is a clear-cut medical emergency that prevents her participation. In addition to the rights set forth in the American Hospital Association's "Patient's Bill of Rights," (which has also been adopted by the New York City Department of Health) the Pregnant Patient, because she represents TWO patients rather than one, should be recognized as having the additional rights listed below.

---

1. *The Pregnant Patient has the right,* prior to the administration of any drug or procedure, to be informed by the health professional caring for her of any potential direct or indirect effects, risks, or hazards to herself or her unborn or newborn infant which may result from the use of a drug or procedure prescribed for or administered to her during pregnancy, labor, birth, or lactation.

2. *The Pregnant Patient has the right,* prior to the proposed therapy, to be informed, not only of the benefits, risks, and hazards of the proposed therapy but also of known alternative therapy, such as available childbirth education

classes which could help to prepare the Pregnant Patient physically and mentally to cope with the discomfort or stress of pregnancy and the experience of childbirth, thereby reducing or eliminating her need for drugs and obstetric intervention. She should be offered such information early in her pregnancy in order that she may make a reasoned decision.

3. *The Pregnant Patient has the right,* prior to the administration of any drug, to be informed by the health professional who is prescribing or administering the drug to her that any drug which she receives during pregnancy, labor, and birth, no matter how or when the drug is taken or administered, may adversely affect her unborn baby, directly or indirectly, and that there is no drug or chemical which has been proven safe for the unborn child.

4. *The Pregnant Patient has the right,* if Cesarean section is anticipated, to be informed prior to the administration of any drug, and preferably prior to her hospitalization, that minimizing her and, in turn, her baby's intake of nonessential preoperative medicine will benefit her baby.

5. *The Pregnant Patient has the right,* prior to the administration of a drug or procedure, to be informed of the areas of uncertainty if there is NO properly controlled follow-up research which has established the safety of the drug or procedure with regard to its direct and/or indirect effects on the physiological, mental and neurological development of the child exposed, via the mother, to the drug or procedure during pregnancy, labor, birth, or lactation—(this would apply to virtually all drugs and the vast majority of obstetric procedures).

6. *The Pregnant Patient has the right,* prior to the administration of any drug, to be informed of the brand name and generic name of the drug in order that she may advise the health professional of any past adverse reaction to the drug.

7. *The Pregnant Patient has the right* to determine for herself, without pressure from her attendant, whether she will accept the risks inherent in the proposed therapy or refuse a drug or procedure.

8. *The Pregnant Patient has the right* to know the name and qualifications of the individual administering a medication or procedure to her during labor or birth.

9. *The Pregnant Patient has the right* to be informed, prior to the administration of any procedure, whether that procedure is being administered to her for her or her baby's benefit (medically indicated) or as an elective procedure (for convenience, teaching purposes, or research).

10. *The Pregnant Patient has the right* to be accompanied during the stress of labor and birth by someone she cares for, and to whom she looks for emotional comfort and encouragement.

11. *The Pregnant Patient has the right,* after appropriate medical consultation, to choose a position for labor and for birth which is least stressful to her baby and to herself.

12. *The Obstetric Patient has the right* to have her baby cared for at her bedside if her baby is normal and to feed her baby according to her baby's needs rather than according to the hospital regimen.

13. *The Obstetric Patient has the right* to be informed in writing of the name of the person who actually delivered her baby and the professional qualifications of that person. This information should also be on the birth certificate.

14. *The Obstetric Patient has the right* to be informed if there is any known or indicated aspect of her or her baby's care or condition which may cause her or her baby later difficulty or problems.

15. *The Obstetric Patient has the right* to have her and her baby's hospital medical records complete, accurate, and legible and to have their records, including Nurses' Notes, retained by the hospital until the child reaches at least the age of majority, or, alternatively, to have the records offered to her before they are destroyed.

16. *The Obstetric Patient,* both during and after her hospital stay, has the right to have access to her complete hospital medical records, including Nurses' Notes, and to receive a copy upon payment of a reasonable fee and without incurring the expense of retaining an attorney.

It is the obstetric patient and her baby, not the health professional, who must sustain any trauma or injury resulting from the use of a drug or obstetric procedure. The observation of the rights listed above will not only permit the obstetric patient to participate in the decisions involving her and her baby's health care, but will also help to protect the health professional and the hospital against litigation arising from resentment or misunderstanding on the part of the mother.

Endorsed by the International Childbirth Education Association
For a complimentary copy send a stamped, self-addressed
envelope to: Committee on Patient's Rights, Box 1900,
New York, NY 10001.

Birth Alternatives

My husband and I stood on our own at great inconvenience and stress at a time when we needed comfort and support. I went to a very good but conventional doctor near home for prenatal checkups until the last trimester. Then, much to the chagrin of my doctor (though she'd agreed to it at first, thinking I'd change my mind), I began seeing the nurse-midwives at a hospital an hour from home.

It turned out that I needed a great deal of medical intervention anyway. However, our trouble was worth it, because they were very supportive of nursing. They brought the baby to me regularly even when I was too drugged from general anesthesia to be able to nurse. I was encouraged to nurse when I was able, even though I had a uterine infection and was being given antibiotics intravenously. They also encouraged as much involvement of my husband as was possible, even to his being present during the Cesarean.

Taking a tour of hospital facilities and birth centers in your area can help you decide where you want to give birth. In some areas of the country, a woman can choose from many established alternatives: hospital, midwife service as part of a standard OB/GYN department, an independent birth center, or birth at home. In other regions, it may be a struggle just to insure that you will be able to have the person of your choice with you during labor and birth.

Your local childbirth education group is a good source of information about birth alternatives in your area, but assume the responsibility for investigating all options for yourself. One woman's ideal birth setting may be unsuitable for another for a wide variety of reasons. Do not enroll for the first childbirth-class series you encounter. Obtain sample brochures, and attend any public film showings organizations provide. If possible, call an instructor to discuss class content and approach. In general, the best classes are those given by a community-based, consumer organization that does not rely on referrals from hospitals and doctors for its existence. Too often, classes sponsored by hospitals only discuss their own routines, skirting the issues of whether their practices are necessarily in the best health interests of mothers and babies. The same often holds true for the course taught in the physician's office by someone in the doctor's employ. You are prepared for *their* way of handling birth, but not encouraged to style your own.

Hospitals are in strong competition with one another for maternity clients these days, due to falling birth rates and pressures from regional health agencies to close units with fewer than 1,500 births annually. These conditions make excellent opportunities for the educated consumer to accomplish changes in the routine care offered to laboring women.

The Mothers' Center in Hicksville, Long Island, encourages parents to use their questionnaire when taking a hospital tour. If certain questions cannot be answered by the individual conducting the tour, write the hospital administrator for clarification.

Hospital Tour Questionnaire

Is It Your Hospital Policy To:

		YES	NO
1.	Routinely complete any forms before admission?	___	___
	How many are done in the hospital, and when?	___	___
2.	Routinely send out prenatal patient information package?	___	___

By what mechanism, and when is it given to the woman? _____

3. Routinely inform patients of a current billing
   schedule in writing?   ___ ___
   Can this be obtained by a telephone request for those
   who are not yet registered?   ___ ___

4. Routinely offer prenatal courses in:
   a. prepared childbirth? What type of
      instruction?   ___ ___
   b. baby care?   ___ ___
   c. other courses—please specify? _____

   What is the cost for each?   a. _____ b. _____ c. _____
   Are they taught by staff or
   an outside instructor?   a. _____ b. _____ c. _____
   Are the courses evaluated?   a. _____ b. _____ c. _____
   When are they given?   a. _____ b. _____ c. _____
   May fathers attend?   a.._____ b. _____ c. _____

   What percentage of the women who delivered attended
   prepared childbirth classes?   _____

   What percent of that total were able to deliver vaginally?   _____

   Do you offer a refresher course for multiparas?   _____
   How many sessions?   _____
   What topics do they include? _____

5. Routinely offer a tour of facilities including:
   a. labor and delivery suites?   ___ ___
   b. postpartum floor?   ___ ___
   c. newborn nursery?   ___ ___

   Who may have a tour of the facilities? _____

6. Routinely offer the professional services of a
   nurse-midwife?   ___ ___
   Are there any midwives as part of your staff?   ___ ___

YES   NO

7. Have a lounge adjacent to delivery suites for fathers
   or one companion of choice?   ____   ____
   If no, where does the companion wait for the time he/she
   is separated from the patient? _____

8. Routinely separate mother and father during
   preparation period?   ____   ____

9. Routinely remove all personal belongings?   ____   ____
   What is done with them? _____

10. If the doctor does not leave instructions, who may
    perform rectal and vaginal examinations:
    a. Nurse?   ____   ____
    b. Intern?   ____   ____
    c. Other—please specify? _____

11. Have an early labor lounge?   ____   ____
    If no, what happens to the women who live a
    distance from the hospital and arrive early? _____

12. Have fetal monitoring machines?   ____   ____
    If so, is it routinely required of all patients?   ____   ____
    a. internal?   ____   ____
    b. external?   ____   ____

    Are IVs used routinely?   ____   ____

13. Give permission to remain ambulatory during:
    a. early labor?   ____   ____
    b. advanced labor?   ____   ____

14. Allow labor, delivery, and recovery in:
    a. same room?   ____   ____
    b. same bed?   ____   ____

15. Give permission to have coach of choice present:
    a. supportive person certified in prepared
       childbirth method?   ____   ____
    b. supportive person uncertified in prepared
       childbirth method?   ____   ____
    If yes, what, if any, type of approval is necessary?_____

YES   NO

16. Allow coach to be present: Certified   Uncertified
    a. in labor room?   ___ ___   ___ ___
    b. in delivery room?   ___ ___   ___ ___
    c. in recovery room?   ___ ___   ___ ___
    d. at C-section?   ___ ___   ___ ___
    e. if delivery occurs before
       course is completed?   ___ ___   ___ ___

17. Have someone remain with the woman during an
    unprepared birth?   ___ ___
    If yes, who? _____
    Number of labor rooms _____
    Number of delivery rooms _____
    Nursing staff for days _____ evenings _____ nights _____

18. Give permission to have a hushed room, dim lights,
    and warm bath for the child during delivery?   ___ ___

19. Have an anesthesiologist for obstetrics on the
    premises 24 hours daily?   ___ ___
    If available, must patient pay regardless of use?   ___ ___

20. Use restraints routinely during a prepared birth?   ___ ___

21. Allow immediately following delivery:
    a. mother to hold infant?   ___ ___
    b. mother to nurse on delivery table?   ___ ___

22. Allow pictures to be taken in the:
    a. delivery room?   ___ ___
    b. postpartum room?   ___ ___

23. Routinely use:
    a. silver nitrate?   ___ ___
    b. other eyedrops—please specify? _____

YES   NO

24. Allow a 45-minute recovery period immediately
    following delivery as a family unit?   ____ ____
    If no, how long can the family
    unit remain together? _____

25. How soon after birth is the infant examined by a
    pediatrician? _____

26. What is the hospital policy concerning infant illness
    and death:
    a. in a prepared birth? _____
    b. in a nonprepared birth? _____

27. Permit rooming-in:
    a. complete?   ____ ____
    b. modified?   ____ ____
    c. for what hours? _____

28. What are the visiting hours for fathers or one
    companion? _____
    a. rooming-in patients? _____
    b. all patients? _____

29. Permit demand feeding of infant (if not
    rooming-in):
    a. bottle feeding?   ____ ____
    b. breastfeeding?   ____ ____

30. Have available experienced advice for breast-
    feeding mothers?   Unaware ____   ____ ____

31. Routinely offer postnatal courses (in
    addition to one-to-one instructions):
    a. on infant care?   ____ ____
    b. on physical and emotional aspects of
       postpartum period?   ____ ____
    c. When are they given?   a. _____ b. _____
    d. May fathers attend?   a. _____ b. _____

32. Have an obstetrical social worker?   ____ ____
    Have an obstetrical psychiatric consultant?   ____ ____
    Have a home care coordinator?   ____ ____

33. Permit a choice in the length of hospitalization?
    a. for mother?   ____ ____
    b. for baby?   ____ ____
    If no, what is the range for length of stay? _____

34. Allow sibling visitation (specify minimum
    age of visitor):
    a. with mother? _____
    b. with baby? _____

35. Allow family meals:
    a. on holidays?   ____ ____
    b. other times?   ____ ____

36. Accept women in labor not registered?   ____ ____
    Under what circumstances (e.g., centimeters
    dilated, census, etc.) _____

37. Have available maternal/fetal transport unit?   ____ ____
    If yes, can mother be accommodated?   ____ ____
    Who can make a request for use? _____

    If no, what is done if a patient calls your
    hospital for transport? _____

38. Routinely ask patients to evaluate your
    maternity services?   ____ ____

39. Have a member of the maternity staff available
    to the public to contact for further information?   ____ ____
    How can this person be reached? _____

Share information obtained on the tour and from other community sources with your doctor or midwife. You may find that the hospital claims all decisions about birth are made by the physician, while the doctor claims some of your preferences can't be satisfied because of hospital policy.

If you are determined, you can usually persuade or negotiate your way to an understanding with your medical attendant. But you must be well informed and sure of your preferences when you seek changes in the routine. If you know that other doctors in the area are cooperating with the specific preferences you have, mention it to your doctor or midwife. If an impasse develops over something that is very important to you, and you have begun your educational process early enough in pregnancy, you will not feel uncomfortable in changing doctors or hospitals. You may even decide to forgo the hospital altogether if it seems rigid and impervious to your needs.

Several national organizations are concerned with extending the option of safe home birth to healthy women. Each maintains a registry of birth attendants and a listing of other publications about the issue of childbirth at home. Conferences and workshops, for parents and professionals, are held in various locations around the country. For schedules and information about home birth in your area contact:

Association for Childbirth at Home, International (ACHI)
6840 Orangethorpe Ave., Suite E
Buena Park, CA 92060
Telephone: (213) 802-1020

National Association of Parents and Professionals for Safe Alternatives in Childbirth (NAPSAC)
National Headquarters
P.O. Box 267
Marble Hill, MO 63764
Telephone: (314) 238-2010

Institute for Childbirth and Family Research
2522 Dana St., Suite 201
Berkeley, CA 94704
Telephone: (415) 849-3665

National Midwives Association
1119 E. San Antonio Ave.
El Paso, TX 79901
Telephone: (915) 533-8142

To find out where there is a midwifery service as part of a hospital OB/GYN department near you, write or call:

American College of Nurse-Midwives
1000 Vermont Ave. NW
Washington, DC 20005
Telephone: (202) 347-5445

Cesarean Birth

It is inevitable that a small percentage of babies must be born by Cesarean section. Cesareans Support, Education, and Concern (C/SEC) of Boston, a Cesarean parents' support group which also performs educational services for medical personnel, publishes a list of guidelines for family-centered Cesareans. It is wise to discuss the manner in which Cesareans are handled at the hospital you have chosen and with the midwife or physician you see for prenatal care. C/SEC notes that parents who look forward to sharing the birth of their baby, to participating actively in labor and birth, and to immediate, intimate contact with their infant at birth and subsequently, often experience great disappointment when a Cesarean must be performed.

Their disappointment at being separated from each other and then from their babies (perhaps at the time when they *most* need to be together for mutual support) and the other fears, angers, hurts, and resentments that accompany an operative delivery are often extremely intense and hard to adjust to. Postpartum, the Cesarean mother has a much more difficult time. The physical pain and limitations of a Cesarean mother are often minimized by the hospital staff as well as by friends and relatives. Members of nursing staffs have readily admitted to C/SEC representatives that they often do not treat the Cesarean mother differently, though she has had *major* surgery.

Emotionally, it is somewhat difficult for a woman who has looked forward to the birth of her infant to accept the fact that she may never be able to experience the event normally. Often a Cesarean baby is taken to the Special Care (or Intensive Care) Nursery for an extended period of time which adds to the mother's depressed state. If she has other children at home, the traditional seven-day stay in the hospital is unusually difficult.

One C/SEC counselor explains:

People who have joined our organization for personal reasons—having had a surprise Cesarean themselves—have subsequently commented on the tremendous importance of education and preparation for this kind of a birth. They, like anyone else, were

I had a Cesarean when I'd wanted a home birth. I hadn't considered the possibility that I'd have complications during delivery. But even before the midwife and doctor agreed, I felt that a Cesarean was indicated. Even so, afterwards I felt a tremendous sense of failure and disappointment. My sense of control over my own body was shaken, and I went through a period where I blamed myself and the doctors. Now, 8½ months later, I don't blame anyone. I look forward to my next delivery and hope it will be normal to make up for this unfortunate experience.

convinced that Cesareans happen to OTHER people. . . . For the past two years I have been receiving letters and phone calls from Cesarean mothers. Invariably, the comment, "If only someone had told me," comes into the discussion. C/SEC guidelines are an attempt to eliminate that phrase, and in so doing, help Cesarean parents relax and enjoy the birth of their infant even under the surrounding surgical conditions.

C/SEC Guidelines

Immediate procedures to expect:

- shaving body in area of surgery,
- antiseptic painting of abdomen,
- insertion of catheter to drain bladder,
- possible cardiac monitor,
- insertion of intravenous apparatus into arm, and
- initiation of anesthesia (through intravenous or by mask for general anesthesia; into or around spinal column for regional anesthesia, such as an epidural).

Facts about Cesareans:

1. The catheter may not be removed for 24 to 48 hours. This is one procedure that many Cesarean mothers complain about. Many find it extremely uncomfortable for that length of time.
2. Intravenous is generally left in for 24 to 48 hours.
3. A screen may be placed directly in front of the mother's face. Some doctors feel this is necessary to create a sterile field; others do not insist upon the screen.
4. The mother can remain awake (spinal Cesareans or epidural anesthesia—acupuncture has even been used for some!) or be given general anesthesia. Many doctors prefer regional anesthesia throughout; however, some use regional until the baby is born and then give a general anesthesia.
5. The entire procedure takes about 45 minutes. The baby is delivered within the first 5 to 10 minutes, and the remaining time is for the closing (suturing) of the incision. (Some mothers have been very uncomfortable because of allergic reactions to suturing material. Ask doctor to check on this.)
6. Cesarean mothers can be successful nursing mothers, even if it happens that getting started is slower than usual.
7. The baby may be brought to the Special Care Nursery for an observation period. (Many mothers become frantic when told that the baby has gone to the SCN, not

realizing that this is just a general hospital procedure and is done even when the baby is perfectly healthy.)

8. Mother will go to the recovery room following the Cesarean.

9. Pain medication is available following the operation, and may be necessary for several days. (Flatulence is often a problem after a Cesarean.)

10. Mothers are usually required to get up and walk the day after the operation and are encouraged to do so several times each day. (Basic exercises are included in chapter 3.)

11. Rooming-in is possible. The Cesarean mother will need help caring for the baby in the first few days: lifting the baby, positioning the baby, changing the baby from one breast to the other, and so on.

12. It is not uncommon to have a fever after surgery, but mother and baby do not necessarily have to be separated.

13. The average hospital stay is six to seven days. The stitches or clamps are usually removed at about the fifth day. (Some doctors use dissolvable stitches.)

14. At home, mother should refrain from lifting, housework, and driving for several weeks. She has had major surgery and should be treated accordingly.

15. Mothers generally report that they feel physically back-to-normal anywhere from one week to six months following the operation. Obviously, other factors are involved.

16. The scar fades in most cases. If a repeat Cesarean is done, the same incision is used. The nutrition of the mother is important in promoting good healing.

17. Vaginal deliveries are sometimes possible after having had a Cesarean. Even when a subsequent birth is almost certain to be a repeat C-section, some doctors will allow a woman to go into labor beforehand.

18. Babies born by section are in a statistically higher risk category for hyaline membrane, respiratory distress, and other problems.

19. One other thing that might be mentioned is that during some Cesareans, there is little talk in the operating room; during others, doctors discuss the previous nights sports events. This may be to relieve tension, but in either case, mothers have felt uncomfortable.

Cesarean Birth Preferences

The following have been requested by Cesarean parents, and *all* or *some* of the answers have been yes, depending on the doctor and hospital. Positive responses to these requests make the Cesarean experience more pleasant and meaningful, and more family centered (We have noted that the attitude of the couple involved is important. "My husband and I want to be together during the birth. We know of couples who have been and want suggestions to realize this goal." This approach nets better results than, "Is it okay for my husband to be with me?")

WE WOULD LIKE:

- to be together for the birth of our baby. ("If this is the only way our baby can be born, please let us witness it together.")
- to have the screen removed. There is really very little of the incision that can be viewed, but at least the *baby* can be seen.
- to have a low, cervical ("bikini") incision performed. The scar does not show, and with this type of incision, some feel there is a better chance for a future vaginal delivery.
- to remain awake during the entire procedure.
- to nurse the baby on the operating table. This *is* possible in many cases and is easier than later when anesthesia has begun to wear off.
- to hold the baby or at least see it, or perhaps the father can hold it if mother is unable. Note: Often the baby is whisked away with hardly a glance for mother, even when it is quite healthy. Some C/SEC mothers have had to yell, "I want to see that baby again!"
- to be together in the recovery room.
- to have my baby judged on its own merit and to shorten or eliminate the time spent in SCN if baby is healthy.
- to room-in with help from the staff, which, as many mothers attest, helps take the focus off the physical pain and onto that little bundle—a real recovery boost.
- to have an electrically operated bed.
- to have a relative or friend be allowed to stay to help with the care of the baby when the husband is not available. This helps the nursing staff, too!
- to have a Cesarean roommate. It can be quite discouraging to have a roommate popping in and out of bed right after her delivery.
- to visit the SCN if my baby is there.
- to see my other children while I am hospitalized.

Conclusions

The health of the mother and baby is first and foremost. However, the parents' emotional health is also of utmost importance and must be considered. Being able to share the birth of their infant, even when it is by Cesarean, is of extreme importance to many couples. (Fathers are all-too-often forgotten; the concerns they feel when they sit alone while their wives are being operated on, and listening to other men talk about how great it was to be in the delivery room, can be very upsetting.) The women who have been in touch with C/SEC want to feel that their childbirth experience is a beautiful and meaningful one, too, and with the help and understanding of childbirth instructors and health professionals, this can be more easily realized. The Cesarean delivery can then be an event to be looked forward to—*the birth of a baby*, rather than an operation, a lonely, frightening experience as it all too often has been viewed.

For further information; or to contact a C/SEC-affiliated group near you, write:

C/SEC
15 Maynard Rd.
Dedham, MA 02026

For a brochure about their 35-minute slide/tape presentation, "Having a Cesarean Is Having a Baby," write:

C/SEC
114 Boston St.
Salem, MA 01970

Postpartum

The postpartum period begins immediately after the placenta detaches from the wall of your uterus and is expelled (third stage of labor). Depending on the factors being considered, the postpartum period can last from two weeks to two years.

Most textbooks talk about a postpartum recovery period of six weeks, and that is the time when most obstetricians schedule the postpartum checkup. Six weeks is the traditional amount of time women are advised to abstain from sexual relations after childbirth. Six weeks has been assumed to be the time by which your internal organs return to their prepregnancy size, shape, and position in your body. Many women believe they should be back to their prepregnancy weight and dress size by the six-week checkup.

None of these ideas are necessarily true. How long your body takes to adjust to not being pregnant anymore depends on what you do with it. Breast-feeding your baby, for instance, prolongs some aspects of being pregnant—like elevated levels of certain hormones and, for some women, absence of menstrual cycles. A faithfully carried out program of exercise for the pelvic floor muscles (see chapter 3) may mean you can resume intercourse pleasurably within two or three weeks. A sensible eating plan that meets your needs for nutrients (to insure good healing of the placental site or surgical incisions, to insure an adequate supply of high-quality breast milk, and to provide enough energy so you can enjoy caring for your new baby) usually does not result in sudden weight loss. On the other hand, the mother who breast-feeds, eats correctly, and exercises may find herself in a better state of health after having a baby than she was before she became pregnant. She will be taking care of her body from the inside out, creating a foundation of health upon which all other physical considerations (skin, hair, shape, and weight) are based.

Your Body

One could think of the postpartum period as pregnancy in reverse. The uterus, in a process called involution, diminishes in size ½ inch a day until ten days after birth when it can no longer be felt above the pubic bone. Immediately after birth, the uterus feels like a solid mass of tissue about the size of a grapefruit. It should stay tightly contracted in the hours and days after birth so that the place where the placenta was attached does not leak excess blood, causing a postpartum hemorrhage. Breast-feeding your baby on demand is the most effective way to insure that the uterus stays contracted. When the baby suckles, the stimulation of your nipple triggers the release of hormones which cause the uterus to contract. If you have your baby in the hospital, medication to cause uterine contractions will be offered routinely. The breast-feeding mother who has access to her baby day and night will not need to take these drugs. The breakdown of uterine tissue no longer needed in the nonpregnant state, is accomplished by these contractions plus the activity of enzymes.

You can expect to have a discharge similar to menstrual flow for several weeks after birth. Called *lochia,* its color is an index to the process of healing at the placental site. Starting out bright red, it becomes brownish, then clear, and finally ceases altogether. If you should have a resumption of bright red bleeding after passing that phase or a sudden increase in the amount of flow, contact your midwife or physician at once. Often, just curtailing your activities for a day or two will solve the problem. If not, your medical consultant will want to determine the reason for the renewed bleeding.

Once the flow of lochia ceases, your menstrual cycles are likely to be suppressed for several months if you are

I healed very rapidly after birth, and within a few days my bleeding had ceased completely. The soreness and swelling disappeared quite soon, and in a very short time I was swimming at the lake with my 3-week-old daughter sleeping in the shade in her carriage.

Emotionally and psychologically, this was a most enjoyable pregnancy. Although I'm sure there are numerous reasons for this, a major factor, I'm certain, was my superior diet and high protein intake. My nerves were calm, my energy flowed, and I felt tranquil and very happy.

breast-feeding and not offering any other liquids or solids to the baby. Current theories suggest that complete breastfeeding keeps your hormones at levels almost as high as pregnancy, so your ovaries do not release eggs and you do not menstruate. However, the amount of breastfeeding required by an individual mother to suppress ovulation is widely variable. Some women have no menstrual periods until they stop nursing; others menstruate within weeks after birth even though they nurse 10 to 12 times a day.

Unless you are willing to conceive again soon after this birth, it is risky to depend on breastfeeding alone as a contraceptive. Many women are turning to barrier methods of contraception (diaphragm, foam, or condom) or the newer cervical mucus assessment methods rather than taking the pill or having an IUD inserted.

The IUD was irritating and caused excessive bleeding. I absolutely will not consider the pill, because it interferes with the body chemistry. In fact, artificial methods have become abhorrent to both Jim and me. We searched and found the Natural Family Planning program which is based on the use of a combination of natural signs of fertility: ovulation signs (vaginal mucus) and temperature. This program was proven to be the best for us because it is, again, based on the natural.

Many researchers are now reporting serious complications due to the pill and the IUD which did not appear in earlier studies. It is now known, for instance, that the pill alters much more than the menstrual cycle: It changes a woman's entire body in ways that can be damaging over years of use. The IUD is being implicated in numerous deaths and serious pelvic infections requiring major surgery to correct.

For women looking forward to fulfilling years with their children and mates, the ever-increasing risks associated with both of these forms of contraception are no longer acceptable. Barbara and Gideon Seaman's book, *Women and the Crisis in Sex Hormones* (New York: Rawson Associates Publishers, 1977), documents these findings and discusses contemporary alternatives to these forms of birth control.

Other changes to expect in the first few days after giving birth:

- pelvic floor and abdominal wall will be very slack—it took nine months and the stress of labor to stretch your skin and muscles to this extent, so be patient with yourself as you undertake toning exercise for these areas;
- increased urination, perspiration, and thirst—fluid stored in circulation and tissues during pregnancy is no longer needed, but you become thirsty as your breasts begin to secrete milk;
- breasts become fuller, heavier, warm, and tender—milk ducts are filling with milk in response to your infant's suckling; this usually subsides in a day or two as your supply adapts to the baby's demand;
- an episiotomy, if done, may be swollen, sore, and/or itchy as it begins to heal—Kegels plus sitz baths at home help

speed the healing process as does maintaining a high-quality diet;

- hemorrhoids (varicose veins of the anus) may result from strain during birth—you may hold back bowel movements because of pain or fear of pain, causing constipation, but a stool softener prescribed by your midwife or physician or mineral oil taken before going to bed will ease elimination;

- need to rest—giving birth, experiencing these drastic changes in your body, and assuming full-time responsibility for baby care means you need to pamper yourself as much as possible in the early postpartum days. You nap when baby naps, eat good food prepared by someone else, and tell friends and family you will call them when you are ready for visitors. Keep your baby next to you in bed so you don't have to keep getting up to nurse or change diapers. Let someone else take care of the house and errands for a week or so, and try to have your mate take a vacation at this time so you both can get accustomed to your new family member and spend time alone together. Try to keep time for each other no matter how hectic life may seem right now. These early months pass quickly but can disrupt your relationship as a couple (see chapter 6).

Postpartum Depression

Coping with the inevitable stresses that come with having a new baby in the household becomes easier with each subsequent child. Knowing what to expect from the newborn, having certain baby care routines established, gaining expertise in breastfeeding, making realistic appraisals of your figure and energy levels for a few months postpartum, and understanding how your mate can participate in the baby's care are valuable stores of information. Unfortunately, most people have to live through these experiences in order to attain the know-how.

The tendency in pregnancy is to focus almost exclusively on preparing for the birth itself. Awareness of how your life will be different after the baby arrives is harder to imagine if this is your first pregnancy. Nobody can tell you exactly which changes will occur in your life, but you and your mate must discuss and plan for the obvious ones so that you can enjoy your new baby to the fullest and have time for each other apart from meeting the needs of the baby.

Postpartum depression is much more common in women who have thought little about the realities of caring for their infants and whose birth experiences have been less fulfilling than they had anticipated, usually because intervention in the birth became necessary; or because they had mistaken impressions about the enormous physical experiences involved in giving birth. Depression is usually mild or nonexistent in women for whom childbirth and breastfeeding are self-confirming, personally strengthening life experiences. They can only be so when the mother's needs, physical and emotional are met during pregnancy, birth, and postpartum. Improving the experience of childbearing for all women means reorienting priorities in maternity care toward health maintenance and respect for the healthy woman's body.

As women assume more responsibility for the type of prenatal and obstetrical care they receive, changes in birth practices affecting all women can be, must be, brought about.

I want to be the perfect mother but I think I've overdone it. Eight and a half months after our child's birth, my husband and I have virtually not gone out or been alone together. The strain is beginning to show: I am irritable and jumpy a great deal. Because I waited so long to have a child, I felt I could or should give it all my time. But this is unrealistic. I need time for my husband and for myself to be able to be a good mother when I'm with the child.

Recommended Reading

Annas, George J. *The Rights of Hospital Patients.* New York: E. P. Dutton and Co., 1976.

Arms, Suzanne. *Immaculate Deception: A New Look at Women and Childbirth in America.* Boston: Houghton Mifflin Co., 1975.

Bean, Constance. *Labor and Delivery: An Observer's Diary, What You Should Know About Today's Childbirth.* Garden City, New York: Doubleday and Co., 1977.

Boston Women's Health Book Collective. *Our Bodies, Ourselves.* Rev. 2nd ed. New York: Simon and Schuster, 1976.

Bradley, Robert A., *Husband-Coached Childbirth.* New York: Harper and Row, 2nd ed., 1975.

Donovan, Bonnie. *The Cesarean Birth Experience: A Practical, Comprehensive, and Reassuring Guide for Parents and Professionals.* Boston: Beacon Press, 1977.

Haire, Doris. *The Cultural Warping of Childbirth.* Milwaukee: ICEA, 1973.

Hazell, Lester. *Birth Goes Home.* Seattle: Catalyst Publishing Co., 1974.

Hazell, Lester. *Commonsense Childbirth.* New York: Berkeley Publishing Corp., 1976.

Jacobson, Edmund, M.D. *You Must Relax.* New York: McGraw-Hill, 1962.

Kippley, Sheila. *Breastfeeding and Natural Child Spacing: The Ecology of Natural Mothering.* Rev.ed. New York: Harper and Row Publishers, 1974.

Montagu, Ashley. *Life before Birth.* New York: New American Library, 1977.

Noble, Elizabeth. *Essential Exercises for the Childbearing Year: A Guide to Health and Comfort Before and After Your Baby Is Born.* Boston: Houghton Mifflin Co., 1976.

Raphael, Dana. *The Tender Gift: Breastfeeding.* New York: Schocken Books, 1976.

Rich, Adrienne. *Of Woman Born: Motherhood As Experience and Institution.* New York: Bantam Books, 1977.

Rugh, Roberts and Shettles, Landrum B. *From Conception to Birth: The Drama of Life's Beginnings.* New York: Harper and Row Publishers, 1971.

Seaman, Barbara. *Free and Female: The Sex Life of the Contemporary Woman.* New York: Fawcette World Library, 1973.

Seaman, Barbara, and Seaman, Gideon, M.D. *Women and the Crisis in Sex Hormones.* New York: Rawson Associates Publishers, 1977.

Shaw, Nancy Stoller. *Forced Labor: Maternity Care in the United States.* Elmsford, New York: Pergamon Press, 1974.

Sousa, Marion. *Childbirth at Home.* Englewood Cliffs, New Jersey: Prentice-Hall, 1976.

Stewart, David, and Stewart, Lee, eds., *Twenty-First Century Obstetrics Now.* 2 vols. Chapel Hill, North Carolina: NAPSAC, 1977.

Tanzer, Deborah. *Why Natural Childbirth?* Garden City, New York: Doubleday, 1972.

Thevenin, Tine. *The Family Bed: An Age Old Concept in Childrearing.* Minneapolis: Tine Thevenin, 1976.

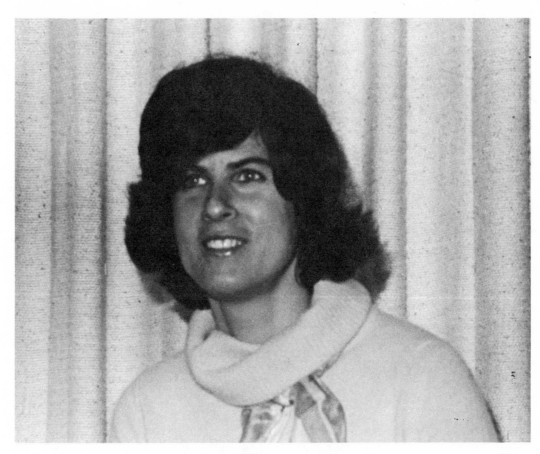

Lynne M. Brody, M.D., practices psychiatry and child psychiatry in Briarcliff Manor, New York. Mother of an active two-year-old boy, she lists nutrition as her chief hobby.

Dr. Brody graduated from New York University School of Medicine, completed an internship in pediatrics at Cedars-Sinai Medical Center, Los Angeles, and a residency in psychiatry and a fellowship in child psychiatry at Albert Einstein College of Medicine in the Bronx, New York.

Her interest in breastfeeding stems from her own experience with nursing. She serves as an advisor to several childbirth and parenting organizations.

5
Breastfeeding:
Completing the Maternity Cycle

Part I

Meeting the Needs of Mother and Baby   by: Lynne M. Brody, M.D.

The physical birth of an infant creates a physically separate individual, but the newborn is still totally dependent on her mother or a substitute to meet both physical and emotional needs. The newborn infant needs to be held close, to smell, feel the warmth, and hear the heartbeat of her mother. She needs to suck, to touch and be touched, and to have eye contact. In addition, she needs a consistent loving relationship with one person, who can offer her security, adapt to her changing needs, and gradually introduce her to the outside world.

The first few years of extrauterine life are ones of extremely rapid development. Before the infant has reached one year, she will have more than tripled her birth weight, be sitting, crawling, standing, and beginning to walk. She will also know who her mother is, feel more comfortable in her presence, recognize others as strangers, and begin to sense her own separateness from her mother.

During this period of unusually rapid physical and emotional development, the child requires an abundance of both nutritional and emotional supports. Nursing, an intimate loving relationship between two human beings, is uniquely designed to meet the nutritional, immunologic, allergic, and emotional needs of the infant, as well as the emotional and physical needs of the mother.

While breast-feeding my baby I had feelings like those I experienced as a teenager when I first fell in love—the excitement of seeing the one you love, waiting for him/her to appear—I couldn't wait for the baby to wake up.

Nursing and the Career-Oriented Mother

The mother over thirty often has a well-established career and wants to keep it, and to her, nursing and full-time motherhood, even for a short time, seems a great disadvantage. She probably enjoys her work and finds it rewarding, and doubts that staying home would offer her any comparable rewards. She may not want to lose her job, her seniority, and the sense of being liberated, or she may fear that she will be too bored at home.

For some mothers, having to be available to an infant most of the time may be seen as a disadvantage of breastfeeding. For those mothers who will nurse only with resentment, bottle feeding offers a better solution. Every

I had to go back to work six weeks after my son was born. At first I came home at lunchtime to nurse him; later I found a baby-sitter near work and nursed him there. It worked out very well.

135

woman, however, even the most career-oriented, should at least consider nursing and what it offers to her child and herself.

The Emotional Needs of the Infant

During the nine months of intrauterine life, the infant has become accustomed to the warmth, smell, heartbeat, and rhythm of the mother. So, after being expelled into a strange world, the baby naturally feels most comfortable and secure in recognizing the familiar scent, heartbeat, and warmth she was used to.

At birth and in the first few postpartum months, the infant is primarily attuned to her own inner feelings and sensations. At first she is only awake briefly, and only in these wakeful moments can she be introduced to the world beyond her inner sensations: to her sensations at the surface of her body and then to her mother. The infant learns about her outer boundaries by feeling her skin against her mother's, with its warmth and softness. She also feels the pressure as she is being held. She learns about mother in repeatedly smelling, being with, and seeing her, particularly her face.

The infant can only look beyond her inner self if her instinctual needs for food and freedom from tension are met. If these are met, with adequate sucking, food, and security, the infant learns to expect her mother's presence and to enjoy this first human relationship. As her needs are continually being met by mother, she begins to believe that she and her mother are really one.

In *The Psychological Birth of the Human Infant* (New York: Basic Books, 1975), Margaret Mahler concludes that "as neurological processes and motor development progress, the infant begins to distance herself physically from her mother, becomes aware of their separateness, learns to cope with it, and establishes an identity of her own, thereby attaining her psychological birth." The infant can only cope with the separateness and become a separate individual psychologically if she has had one consistent mother or mother substitute available to meet her early dependency needs and offer her security, love, and encouragement.

There have been many studies done which show what happens when the needed ingredients for the psychological development of the infant are not available. In *Scientific American* (200:68-74, 1959), Professor Harry Harlow reported on one classic experiment in which infant monkeys were placed alone with a wire mother with a milk bottle attached and a similar cloth-covered wire without milk.

What can ever compare to that beatific look when your baby's eyes gaze upon you as she nurses? Sometimes, I feel there are just the two of us in this whole world, and each of us desperately needs, wants, and adores the other. Our moments of nursing are sheer bliss.

I nursed our baby girl on demand. She took a little many times a day. I never developed sore nipples (though I didn't prepare my breasts for nursing), and she never got into crying fits.

I couldn't stand to hear her cry when I put her to bed at night, so I overcame my fear of rolling on her and took her into bed with us. I feel that the almost constant contact between newborn and other family members makes a happy, independent baby.

Our baby has traveled long distances and been thrust into noisy, crowded parties, restaurants, and the like—all in near-perfect tranquillity. People have often commented on how good she is, and they still do.

Although the monkeys went to the wire mothers for food, they spent the remainder of time clinging to the cloth mothers. None of these monkeys, however, were later able to develop normal monkey relationships.

Another well-known study by Sally Provence and Rose Lipton, described in *Infants in Institutions: A Comparison of Their Development during the First Year of Life with Family-Reared Infants* (New York: International Universities Press, 1962), showed that infants brought up in institutions, where they had many caretakers and not one consistent mother figure, were unable to make normal human attachments when such relationships were offered in foster homes or with adoptive families.

In her recent book, *Every Child's Birthright: In Defense of Mothering* (New York: Basic Books, 1977), Selma Frailberg writes about her experience with children of mothers who worked and have had a variety of caretakers, either at home or in inadequate day-care centers. She describes the impaired ability of these children to form human relationships, and their poor frustration tolerance, increased aggressive behavior, and poor memory function.

D.W. Winnicott, a British child psychiatrist and author of *The Child, the Family and the Outside World* (London: Penguin Books, 1964), has repeatedly stressed the importance of the emotional availability of the mother figure as crucial to the normal development of the infant and child.

Why Breastfeeding?

A good mother who cares about her infant could meet all of her baby's needs with bottle feeding. She could hold her baby in her arms while feeding, allowing the baby to touch her skin and remaining the primary one to feed and care for her. Breastfeeding, however, not only meets these needs naturally, but usually fulfills certain needs in the mother as well, further encouraging this important loving relationship.

When nursing, the child is held in her mother's arms or cradled in a pillow on her lap, so she can reach her mother's breasts. While sucking, she smells her mother's familiar scent, feels her warmth, and hears her comforting heartbeat. Her cheeks feel her breasts, and her hands are free to touch and explore them or her face. When her eyes are open, she sees her mother, and when she looks up, their eyes meet.

A new mother, particularly one who is bottle-feeding, may see her baby more as a burden than a joy. She feels she has all the work to do—washing diapers, clothes, and preparing formula. Yet, she may feel that anyone can feed the baby. Feeding is seen as one more task to be done,

There is a real difference between breast and bottle feeding for me. This baby always smells so sweet. I think he can feel that he is really loved; the way he holds my hand and looks into my eyes as he nurses makes him extremely cuddly. I think this nursing relationship is one of the reasons I have had no postpartum depression! This time there have been only continued days of joyful companionship with the baby.

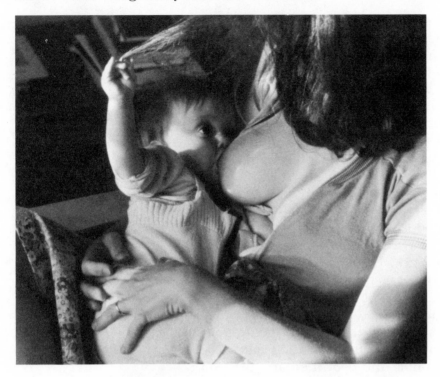

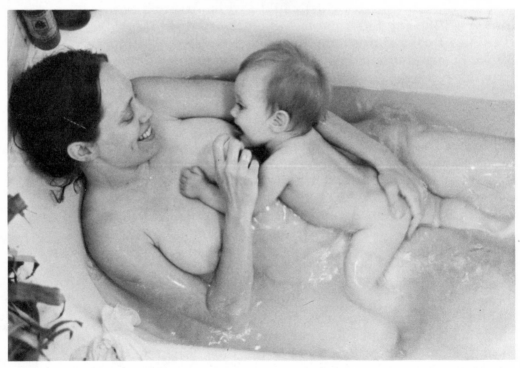

rather than an opportunity for loving.

A mother who breast-feeds will soon feel that *she* herself is needed by her baby, that she has a very special role in nurturing her. This special maternal feeling is partly hormonal, a result of the chemical substances secreted in response to her infant sucking at her breasts. The rest of this important feeling is psychological, feeling loved and needed when her infant looks up so lovingly while feeding, and afterwards, when she falls off to sleep looking blissfully satisfied. These feelings make a mother want to repeat the experience over and over again, and she is unlikely to want to have her baby fed by anyone else. The ease of feeding, with a ready prewarmed supply always available, also makes a mother more likely to take her infant along when she must leave home. This provides a continuity of care in the infant's life.

As nursing continues, the nursing partners become unusually attached to one another, not only child to mother, but mother to child as well. The frequent intimacy helps a mother to empathize with her child, almost feel what her child feels. This makes her exquisitely sensitive to her child's needs, not only for food but also for affection, closeness, stimulation, and later on, for separateness.

Within the loving mother-infant relationship, the infant will find consistency and security and will be able to take risks in learning about her own self and the world beyond. When the time is right, she will be able to separate, because she has already gained enough emotional supplies during the many nursings and hours spent with her mother. She will also feel secure because her sensitive mother will be able to love her for herself as a separate person, knowing this is another of her basic human needs.

This first loving human relationship is critical because it will serve as a model for all of the child's later human relationships.

Nursing Acts as an Antidote to Postpartum Depression

Postpartum depression, the sadness often accompanied by tearfulness and a feeling of uselessness, is rather common to some degree after giving birth in our culture. It is not surprising to see a mother react with sadness when her baby, who has been part of her for nine months is taken away to a nursery and fed by so-called experts, often being told it doesn't matter who feeds her baby, since the baby can't tell anyway. A mother who is nursing her newborn is naturally more likely to feel needed, useful, special, and even vital to her baby's physical and emotional development. She is less likely to become depressed and more likely to remain emotionally available to her infant.

Nursing your baby also offers a unique opportunity to share in an intimate, loving exciting relationship with your

Let's not overlook the physical joy of nursing. It really feels good! So many women react to the thought of nursing with repulsion. How sad. They're missing out on one of womankind's sweetest pleasures.

I love nursing Elise. She cuddles up inside my arms, dreamily closes her eyes, and begins sucking hungrily. Who can describe that delicious sensation as the breast swells with milk and then is so gratefully relieved of its burden by her eager tuggings? It can certainly be a very sensual experience at times.

With the coming of spring, we've been able to take our 17-month-old child for longer walks. Once on the sidewalk, she strides away from us and walks up to strangers, staring up at those who interest her. She seems fearless, and we're sure it's because she nurses on demand and has lots of holding and cuddling. We wanted her to be confident and optimistic, and so far she is.

I had no postpartum depression while nursing; I did have depression with the first baby who was bottle-fed.

own child. You can watch your baby change and grow into a separate person with ideas of her own. You can share with her the many exciting discoveries she makes, and the joy that goes with them: finding out she can move her legs one after the other and crawl, reach the object she wants, stand up and see the world from a new vantage point, and transfer a little stuffed doll from one hand all the way to the other all by herself.

Mutual Sharing of New Experiences

An infant who is part of a loving relationship will find happiness in many parts of the world her mother may not think of: a leaf moving in the wind or a piece of string dangling above her. If her mother is available, she will want to share all these experiences and pleasures with her. Sharing these can be so rewarding to a mother because she is sharing them with someone she loves.

The advantages of breastfeeding may extend long after the child is weaned; the baby who is used to sharing experiences with her mother will want to continue to do so as she gets older. If her mother continues to be available, a child will share her many discoveries and delights.

Mothers of adolescents often complain that they don't really know their children. They say the children don't want to sit down and share their thoughts and feelings with their mother. The sharing has to begin much earlier in the early mother-child relationship, before the child has given up on her mother's availability and sought all sorts of substitutes in peers and teachers. It has to start when mother and child have time together, before nursery school and kindergarten.

The Nutritional Needs of the Infant

In the first months after birth, the newborn infant continues to grow very rapidly, as she did before birth, and therefore continues to have extremely high nutritional needs. While *in utero*, these needs were met by a highly nutritious maternal diet and absorption of the necessary nutrients through the placenta. Now, however, the infant must take these in by herself. She must do this in spite of her rather immature swallowing mechanism and gastrointestinal tract, and therefore needs an easily digestible liquid diet containing a maximal supply of proteins, sugars, fats, vitamins, and minerals.

There are three types of such liquids available: breast milk, commercially prepared formulas, and homemade formulas. Breast milk is specifically designed to meet all

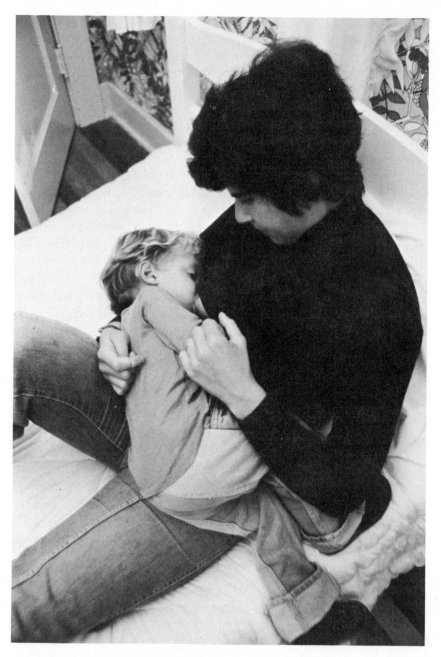

the nutritional needs of the human infant for approximately the first six months of life and does so without potentially hazardous additives and preservatives—and also without extra work for mother.

Breast milk supplies all the proteins, sugars, fats, vitamins, and minerals the human infant requires. They are specifically designed to favor the rapid brain and central nervous system development the newborn infant undergoes. Cow's milk is rather different from human milk in composition, perhaps designed to meet the rapid early bone development evidenced in a calf. Commercial formulas, most of which are made from a cow's milk base, take this liquid which is so different from human milk and modify it in various ways with dilutions and additions to make a final product which resembles human milk as closely as possible.

The formulas available today contain many elements which have been isolated in breast milk. If and when other vitamins and minerals in breast milk are isolated, they may be added to future formulas. Breast milk, however, contains all these nutrients now, whether they have been isolated or not. Formulas must also be heated during preparation, and this process destroys all enzymes and some other nutrients which are then no longer available to the infant. Finally, it has been found that commercial formulas are frequently contaminated with harmful substances.

The other alternative, a homemade formula, once more poses the difficulty of changing a liquid that is chemically different from human breast milk into one that's similar to it. The base used will probably be cow's milk, goat's milk, or soy milk, the final product is likely to be free of preservatives and contaminants, and the added nutrients can be from natural sources. However, it all involves more work and still can be only second best nutritionally.

The Efficiency of Breast Milk

The protein of breast milk, primarily lactalbumin, is digested with almost 100-percent efficiency, due to its small, soft curd. Cow's milk formulas are digested only half as well. This means that the breast-fed infant need take in only half as many calories as she would have to if she were fed a cow's milk formula. Further, she only takes in half the volume of liquid, which in turn, means less work for her immature kidneys.

The sugar in breast milk is lactose, which creates an acidic gastrointestinal tract. This acidity encourages the growth of favorable bacteria, which synthesize B vitamins which are needed and utilized by the infant. It also discourages the growth of pathogenic bacteria that often cause diarrhea. As a result, the breast-fed infant suffers from less diarrhea and diaper rash. The acidity also enhances the absorption of calcium, phosphorus, and vitamin C— nutrients required by the growing infant.

The fats and fatty acids in breast milk include those specifically needed for brain and spinal cord development. These are not available in cow's milk and formulas which have a rather different fat content. Another difference is that breast milk is higher in cholesterol than other formulas which use vegetable oils. At a time when high cholesterol levels are being linked to increasing cardiac and other circulatory system diseases, some formula companies have stressed the value of the vegetable oil content of their products. The vegetable fat content of formulas may, in the long run, turn out to be a disadvantage. First, the fats added to the skimmed cow's milk base are often saturated, such as coconut or cottonseed oil, rather than unsaturated. Second, studies performed on animals suggest that the body may need an early exposure to cholesterol in order to develop mechanisms for its metabolic breakdown. One could infer from these studies that part of our national problem with high blood cholesterol levels might result in part from the formula feeding in infancy of our present-day adults.

Breast milk is higher than cow's milk in vitamins A, B_6, C, E, and K and also niacin and folic acid. In preparing formulas, some of these vitamins are added so that the preparation will more closely simulate breast milk. Not all, however, are replaced. Only some preparations contain added B_6, and none contain folic acid. Both of these vitamins are necessary in the growth and production of new cells throughout the body. Formulas do not contain vitamin K. It is also not clear how or if the infant's body can utilize the added substances in the same way it can assimilate those naturally occurring in human breast milk.

Rickets, a bone disease most commonly due to a lack of vitamin D, is almost never seen in breast-fed infants before they are weaned. Although vitamin D has until now been thought to be only a fat-soluble vitamin, there are some studies being conducted which suggest that there may be a water-soluble form of vitamin D present in breast milk, preventing nursing babies from getting rickets or milder bone abnormalities as a result of this vitamin's deficiency. Cow's milk does not contain any vitamin D, although the fat-soluble form of it is added to formulas.

One further advantage of breastfeeding is that a mother can increase the nutritional content of her milk by simply ingesting much larger quantities of the nutrients herself. I will go into this in more detail later when I discuss the importance of the nursing mother's nutrition.

When it comes to minerals, once more the content in human milk and cow's milk is different. Human breast milk is higher in iron. Its increased absorption due to the acidic state of the gastrointestinal tract, combined with the mother's own iron stores, is usually enough to maintain an infant's iron level until the baby is six months old. Formulas do add iron, but usually in the form of ferrous sulfate, which is less easily absorbed and also interferes with the absorption of vitamin E.

I was so eager to nurse my last baby, because with my others, I had followed the incorrect advice of my pediatrician and cut back to three nursings a day by the second month, so the baby would "have room for solids that would make her grow up." My completely breast-fed baby has grown at a more rapid rate than the others (higher-quality food), and she has never had a problem with digestion or constipation. Taking care of her has been a pleasure, both physically and emotionally.

On the other hand, cow's milk has much more sodium than breast milk. When an infant is sick and losing water through fever and perspiration or diarrhea, this high sodium content may lead to a condition known as hypernatremia, which can cause brain damage.

Cow's milk is also much higher in calcium and phosphorus. The high phosphorus level in infants sometimes causes an imbalance and lowers the calcium levels to such an extent that tetany (muscle contractions), convulsions, and even death can occur as a result of the abnormally low calcium level. Finally, the maternal diet contains many other minerals, such as zinc, copper, magnesium, and perhaps others not yet identified. These are all necessary for human growth and development, and a mother can make sure her baby gets them by including them in her diet.

Comparison of Human Milk and Cow's Milk*

Composition	Human milk	Cow's milk
Water	87.5%	87.2%
Calories	77	66
Protein:	1.1 gr.	3.5 gr.
Casein	40%	82%
Whey	60%	18%
Fat	4.0 gr.	3.7 gr.
Lactose	6.8 gr.	4.8 gr.
Ash	0.2 gr.	0.7 gr.
Selected minerals:		
Calcium	33 mg.	117 mg.
Phosphorus	14 mg.	92 mg.
Iron	0.1 mg.	trace
Sodium	16 mg.	50 mg.
Potassium	51 mg.	140 mg.
Selected vitamins:		
Vitamin A	240 IU	150 IU
Thiamine	.01 mg.	.03 mg.
Riboflavin	.04 mg.	.17 mg.
Niacin	0.2 mg.	0.1 mg.
Vitamin C	5 mg.	1 mg.

* Figures are for each 100 grams (approximately 3½ ounces).
Sources: *Composition of Foods*, Agricultural Handbook no. 8, 1963, U.S. Department of Agriculture.
Fomon, Samuel S., *Infant Nutrition* (Philadelphia: Saunders, 1967).

Nutrition for the Nursing Mother

To provide her infant with an ample supply of high-quality milk, a mother must eat a varied and nutritious diet, containing adequate amounts of protein, calories, fluids, fats, vitamins, and minerals—just as she did during pregnancy. She needs such a diet to maintain her own health, produce milk, and supply the necessary nutrients to her infant.

Milk production depends on a number of factors. It depends on an adequate maternal blood volume as well as on the hormones released from the pituitary gland at the base of the brain in response to the sucking infant. If a mother's blood volume is inadequate, her body will automatically decrease milk production, using what blood is available to supply her own vital organs: heart, lungs, and brain. This phenomenon is most obvious during hot weather when the mother's body fluids must be replenished often. The blood volume needed by a nursing mother requires an adequate intake of fluids, protein, and calories. Protein is needed to keep the ingested fluids in the bloodstream, and calories are needed so that the protein is available for this purpose and not used up as calories for energy. The mechanisms for maintaining the increased fluid volume are similar to those utilized by the pregnant woman as described in Gail Brewer's book, *What Every Pregnant Woman Should Know* (New York: Random House, 1977).

When the pituitary gland of the nursing mother releases hormones into the bloodstream, they are transported to the mammary glands within the breasts. There they act on cells, causing milk to be produced and made available for the infant. The pituitary gland is highly sensitive to emotions, so when a mother is depressed or upset, it may not release the needed hormones. B-vitamin deficiencies are often associated with mood changes, fatigue, and depression. That's why it is important for a nursing mother to get enough of these vitamins if she is to offer her infant a plentiful milk supply.

A mother who is nursing her baby fully, without giving her supplemental formulas or solids, should continue to eat as she did during pregnancy.

Her diet should be high in protein: meats, fish, eggs, dairy products, beans, and nuts. It should also continue to stress calcium-rich milk and other dairy products. In addition, it should include a wide variety of vegetables, fruits, and whole grains to supply an abundance of vitamins, minerals, and additional protein. It should also include salt to maintain the expanded blood volume and to provide the iodine needed by the thyroid gland, which is producing the hormone thyroxin in large amounts during this period. Iodine is found in both iodized salt and saltwater fish. Lastly, the nursing mother needs to drink a lot of fluids, usually about three quarts a day, depending on the temperature of the season and her activity level.

Nursing Mother's Appetite Expands to Meet Needs

The nursing mother continues to need 500 to 1,000 calories per day more than she did before she was pregnant. If she was well nourished during pregnancy, she will have ten pounds or so stored on her body to sustain nursing for about six months. A healthy nursing mother will have the appetite to eat and drink what she and her baby need. She should meet her hunger and caloric requirements with the least-processed, least-refined, and freshest foods available, since they are highest in nutrients.

A new nursing mother should not worry about weight. First, she will use up an additional 500 to 1,000 calories per day over what she did before she was pregnant. Second, a hungry, undernourished, irritable mother will produce a poor milk supply and a malnourished fussy infant, and the important early mother-child relationship will not be a comfortable one. In addition, it may not be good for a nursing mother to lose weight suddenly, because this further mobilizes her fat supplies, and her milk will then contain higher levels of potentially hazardous chemicals for her infant to ingest.

Once her infant starts to cut down on nursing and begins to eat solid food, the mother's appetite gradually decreases. She will then find that her weight gradually returns to prepregnancy levels, without risk to her own or her infant's physical or emotional health.

Things to Avoid While Nursing

A mother's milk reflects everything in her diet—not only the valuable nutrients, but also less-desirable elements: caffeine, alcohol, drugs, nicotine, additives, pesticides, and industrial hydrocarbons. This does not mean a mother must totally avoid drinking coffee, tea, and alcoholic beverages or stop smoking. It does mean that she should know that what she takes into her body does reach her baby. The concentration of what she ingests is less in her milk than in her own bloodstream, but it is present.

The concerned nursing mother can limit her intake of these known harmful substances. For example, she might substitute decaffeinated coffee and herb teas for regular coffee and caffeine-containing dark teas, drink beer or wine with a lower alcohol content than hard liquor, and limit the number of cigarettes she smokes. Each mother must weigh the advantages and disadvantages that a given substance presents to her and her baby. It is not beneficial to an infant for the mother to give up smoking entirely, if that means the mother is always irritable and emotionally unavailable to the baby.

Some level of almost every drug taken by the mother, both prescription and nonprescription, shows up in breast milk. While some seem to be relatively harmless to the infant, few have been extensively tested. Other drugs do have definite effects on the nursing infant. Some tranquilizers cause restlessness and irritability in the nursing infant. One antitubercular drug, taken over a period of time, can cause mental retardation in the infant. Once more, this does not mean a nursing mother can never take any drugs. She should, however, avoid any drugs she does not absolutely have to take and take those she must only at the recommendation of a physician who knows her condition. He must be aware that she is nursing and must evaluate the possible effect of the drug on her nursing child.

The nursing mother, like the pregnant woman, must be an educated consumer of medical services. Even when a physician prescribes a drug, she should ask why she needs it. Not every sore throat requires antibiotics; for example, those caused by a virus do not. She should also inquire about the necessity of any injections, vaccinations, or office treatments. Even when a drug would cure a symptom, a nursing mother should ask about possible nonmedicinal alternatives: deep-breathing exercises for mild insomnia, a walk in fresh air for headaches, and a talk with an understanding friend or professional when nervous or depressed.

La Leche League International maintains a list of drugs and their effects on the nursing baby. Any L.L.L.I. leader can share their information (all referenced to the medical literature) with you and your physician.

Can Environmental Hazards Contaminate Breast Milk?

Recently, there has been a lot of concern about the possible dangers to the nursing infant of human breast milk containing high levels of DDT and other agricultural pesticides and industrial hydrocarbons. These substances have been shown to cause cancer and other serious disorders in animals and humans. These substances are stored in fat, and when a mother nurses, some of these stores are mobilized, and the toxic substances get into her bloodstream and subsequently into her milk. Infant formulas have been shown to contain lower levels of these toxins, and as a result, some mothers have decided they would be harming their infants unnecessarily by nursing. In a few areas where toxin levels are unusually high, a mother may be warned by her physician and forced into a decision against breastfeeding, but for most of the country, that need not be the answer.

A mother can control the content of her milk to a certain extent. She can decrease her own intake of hydrocarbon pesticides by decreasing her intake of animal fat both before and while nursing. She can avoid fatty cuts of meat and try to get meat from grass-fed, rather than grain-fed animals. Often, such cuts are even less expensive, because with less fat they are tougher. She can also select dairy products which are relatively low in fat, such as skim milk, yogurt, and cottage cheese, and avoid high-fat, low-protein products, such as butter and cream. To make sure she has enough fats in her diet, the nursing mother who is concerned about toxin levels should choose spreads made from 100-percent corn oil or other vegetable oils, cook with vegetable oils, and add nuts to her diet for their natural inner section, or germ. A deficiency of fat can interfere with the absorption of certain vitamins and minerals and may be reflected in skin and hair that looks less than healthy.

The industrial hydrocarbons, known to be harmful, are found primarily in freshwater and saltwater areas close to shore. The nursing mother can avoid eating freshwater fish and that which is from close-lying areas, concentrating on saltwater fish which are not too large and therefore not high in mercury, such as cod and haddock.

Finally, she can avoid strenuous dieting which even further mobilizes fat and toxic substances while nursing. There will be plenty of time for dieting without possible long-term risks to her infant when she is no longer nursing. In *Birthright Denied: The Risks and Benefits of Breastfeeding* (Washington, D.C.: Environmental Defense Fund, 1977), the authors, S.G. Harris and J.H. Highland, cite an example supporting the value of diet in decreasing toxic pesticide residues in human milk. In *Nature et Progres* (4:21-29, Nov.-Dec., 1974), C. Aubert describes a study made in France in which women who ate a primarily vegetarian diet with a high percentage of unsprayed organic foods for six years had less than half the toxic residues present in their milk compared to the milk of women who ate a varied, nonvegetarian diet.

Medical Advantages of Breastfeeding

In addition to emotional and nutritional benefits, nursing offers immunologic protection against disease, decreases the likelihood of allergic reactions, and may prevent obesity in the years to come.

Babies are born with antibodies, the immunity factors against disease, which they received *in utero*. These rapidly lose their effectiveness during the first few months of life, even before the infant's immunologic system is able to produce its own antibodies, leaving her susceptible to infections. The nursing baby, however, receives a continuous supply of immunity factors in her mother's milk, offering her protection against a wide variety of illnesses. During the first year of life, the breast-fed baby has significantly fewer respiratory infections, less diarrhea caused by pathogenic bacteria in the intestinal tract, and fewer infectious illnesses of any type.

Breast-fed infants have few allergic reactions. Allergy to breast milk is unheard of, and mild reactions to something in the mother's diet are rare and eliminated when she eliminates the specific substance from her diet. On the other hand, allergic reactions to cow's milk formulas are frequent, averaging about one in 15. These allergic reactions are often severe with painful cramps, vomiting, diarrhea, and if it continues long enough, malnutrition due to the decreased absorption and loss of nutrients.

These allergic reactions also interfere with the emotional aspects of the early mother-child relationship. The infant who is in constant pain and possibly malnourished is hard to comfort. The new mother will try to quiet her at first, but it all seems in vain after a while. Instead of feeling loved and needed, she may end up feeling disliked and useless. She may find herself either reacting with anger to her irritable infant or spending less and less time with the child, feeling frustrated and bitter after all her futile attempts to comfort the baby. Such early negative interactions, unless there is good supportive intervention, can only set the stage for future difficulties.

Since breast milk readily supplies all the nutrients a full-term nursing infant requires for the first six months or so, solids do not have to be introduced before that time. By six months, the intestinal tract is more mature, and a new food is less likely to be absorbed in such a way as to cause an allergic reaction.

The body chemistry needed to produce an allergic reaction is inherited. It is therefore especially important for an infant to be breast- rather than formula-fed when one or both parents or other close relatives have any allergies, whether to foods, pollens, dust, or animals.

Today, a large percentage of our population is concerned with obesity problems and dieting. It has been found that most fat people have more fat cells than thin people, and that these are created in childhood. One theory suggests that the higher caloric intake of formula-fed babies may cause an increased production of fat cells. Also, bottle-fed babies usually begin to eat solids at an earlier age, and the solids are still higher in calories. Obesity and overeating are also related to eating habits which are learned very early. The mother who bottle-feeds her infant may urge her to finish the entire bottle, and soon, the entire portion of solids set out, rather than allowing the infant to drink and eat only until her thirst and hunger are satisfied.

For the mother, nursing causes the release of pituitary hormones which then cause the uterus to contract, decreasing any likelihood of hemorrhage in the postpartum days. The uterus will also return to its prepregnancy size sooner than that of the nonnursing mother for the same reasons.

Long-term studies have revealed that nursing mothers are less likely to get breast cancer than those who do not nurse, all other genetic and environmental factors being equal.

As for the economics of breastfeeding, it is less expensive than bottle feeding. Although the extra caloric intake of the mother does cost something, this expense is significantly less than buying bottles, sterilizing equipment, formula, and early solids.

Who Can Nurse?

Almost any mother who has just given birth can nurse her newborn baby, and certainly the woman over thirty is no exception. The exceptions are women with highly contagious, untreated cases of tuberculosis or whooping cough or women with a severe terminal illness, such as cancer. In some cases, an infant with a cleft palate or other congenital abnormality or a weak premature infant may not be able to suck, but she can still be given her mother's milk from a tube until ready to nurse. Women who have delivered by Cesarean section can nurse, and so can those who have Rh incompatibilities. Twins as well as prematures can nurse.

Breastfeeding is extremely important for the premature infant, for both nutritional and emotional reasons and has recently been recommended by the American Academy of Pediatrics as the method of choice for feeding them. Nutritionally, the ease of digestibility of breast milk means the baby need not work as hard to take in her required nutrients, and it has also been associated with fewer medical complications for the premature baby. Emotionally, the premature infant will need as much physical contact with her mother as she can get. She needs the warmth and heartbeat she was robbed of too early, and the stimulation she may have had to miss when separated for medical procedures. The mother with a breast infection and the mother who has had breast surgery can usually nurse.

It is very important for the mother to receive clear information and support for her efforts to nurse. The La Leche League can provide counseling, free of charge, for mothers with every type of special nursing situation.

The nursing relationship is unparalleled. It is a relationship designed by nature to best meet both the nutritional and emotional needs of the newborn infant, separate physically, but still totally dependent on another human being. It is a relationship that also offers emotional benefits for the mother which encourage her to remain available and be the constant human contact her baby needs for normal development.

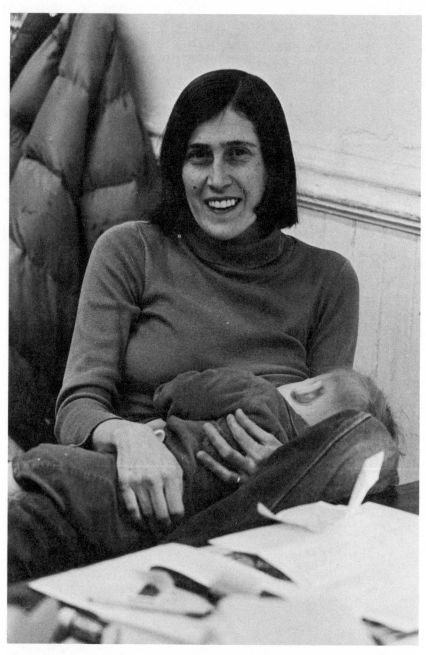

Margot Parsons, a breastfeeding counselor and mother of Heather, 5, and Owen, 8 months, has commented on breastfeeding and mothering for several publications.

A staff member of the Soho Weekly News, she lives with her photographer husband, Rodger, in a Manhattan loft they are renovating.

She is a leader of a New York City mother-to-mother breastfeeding support group for La Leche League International and a founding member of the Cooperative Childbirth Network.

Part II

How to Keep on Breastfeeding— No Matter What Else Happens! by: Margot Pordes Parsons

For many mothers, breastfeeding is hard to separate from the very manner in which they mother. Nursing for these mothers and babies represents an intimate relationship that amounts to far more than the best source of infant nutrition. In some ways, it resembles falling in love, for mother and baby have physical interdependency and long for one another when they are separated. This aspect of the nursing relationship can never be duplicated by a formula company and merchandised. Yet women are advised at almost every turn to stop nursing on the slightest provocation.

Should you find yourself in one of these situations, where you are being advised/pressured to switch your baby to artificial feeding, you will need encouragement to continue to nurse. Herewith a primer of how to keep nursing—no matter what else happens in your life!

I never stop being surprised by people who ask me if breast-feeding isn't too much of a bother now that my baby is almost a year old. Wouldn't a bottle be a more convenient substitute, they ask. I reply that I wouldn't think of sending in a substitute to make love with my husband, so why should I substitute something other than me for my baby?

WHAT IF. . .the hospital interferes with my early attempts to breast-feed?

Breastfeeding seems to follow the birth of a baby naturally. Your body prepares for this sequence by producing colostrum for the newborn and gradually changing to mature milk over the course of the first few days postpartum. In today's hospital, however, this process may be subverted by:

- rigid scheduling of infant feeding on a four-hour schedule,
- a policy of not bringing babies out to nurse during the night,
- the practice of feeding babies glucose water or formula in the nursery despite clear directions to the contrary by the nursing mother,
- the restriction of sucking to a few mintues on each side at each feeding, and
- a lack of competent breastfeeding counselors on the staff.

If the mother has had a Cesarean birth, insensitivity to her desire to breast-feed may take the form of a nurse leaving the baby in a bassinet stationed across the room, rather than placing the baby in the mother's arms and

153

helping her get the baby sucking before leaving.

RECOMMENDATION:

Leave the hospital as soon as possible after you and your baby are examined and found healthy. Shortening the amount of time you are subjected to unnecessary scheduling means you will have your baby to yourself much sooner. Then, as Mary B. Carson (editor) notes in the second edition of her book, *The Womanly Art of Breastfeeding* (Franklin Park, Illinois: La Leche League International, 1963), "Whatever the ups and downs of your hospital stay, when you get your baby home you will be able to nurse him." Get in touch with your local La Leche League group before you give birth. There you can discuss local pediatricians with other nursing mothers and perhaps locate one who will write orders for your baby to be fed on demand, regardless of the routine hospital policy.

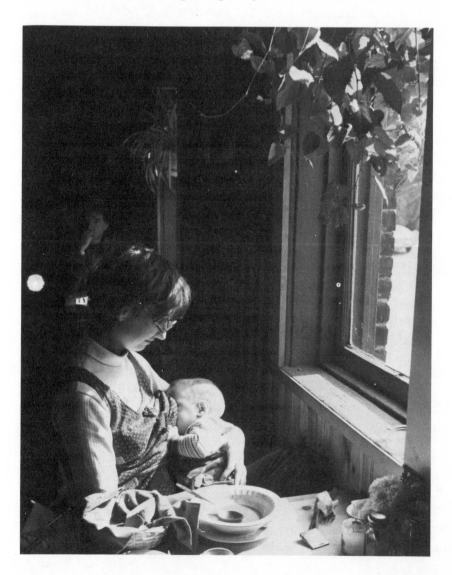

WHAT IF. . .I have a family situation which makes me extremely uncomfortable about nursing?

Many of our mothers attempted to breast-feed and were unsuccessful for numerous reasons. In the United States, only ten percent of mothers are still breast-feeding after the baby is one month old. If the situation requires, excuse yourself from the room when your baby needs to feed and find a private spot. It is much more important for you to nurse your baby than to try to change the ingrained opinions of people who find breastfeeding offensive. Don't let their negative comments influence your decision to nurse. Just do it apart from them or ask the other person to leave.

It was amazing how many people were disturbed by my nursing for more than six months. My husband was great about running interference for us.

RECOMMENDATION:

Before your baby is born, discuss your plans to breast-feed with family members, just to see what their reactions will be. It is important for you to feel comfortable when you nurse in order for your milk to flow easily from your breasts. Attending La Leche League meetings will put you in contact with other mothers who are nursing or who want to find out more about it. Often, you may be the only mother you know who is nursing. It is a help to know other mothers who have done it successfully and on whom you can call if you develop a problem. This is especially valuable when your home-front support is weak.

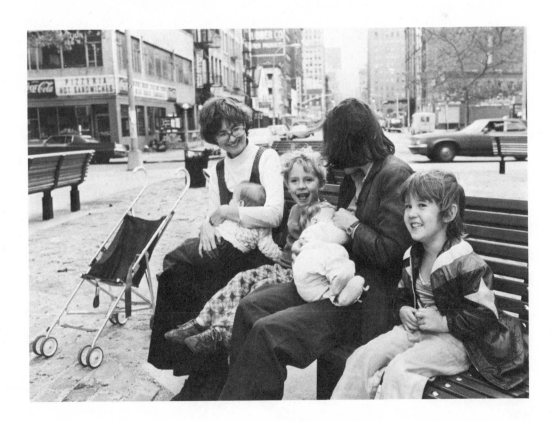

I had no trouble with nursing and did it everywhere—in store lounges, at dinner parties, in the car in parking lots, in class, and in restaurants.

In our work, my husband and I travel a great deal. We could never have continued to work together after the baby came if I hadn't breast-fed. Lugging all that formula, warming it up, and cleaning the bottles afterward would have been too much work for me. I made a point to purchase clothes with two pieces and happily resumed flying trips three weeks after giving birth. No one ever knew I was nursing—not on airplanes, trains, buses, taxis, nor in restaurants, lobbies, conference rooms, or television studios. I never asked anyone's permission—I just went ahead and did it! The baby was so calm and friendly as a result of never having to wait for meals that people everywhere have commented on her good disposition.

WHAT IF. . .I have to travel with my baby?

No matter where you have to go, your baby can go with you! Wearing two-piece garments so you can nurse discreetly is easy. If a long trip is necessary, you will find nursing a comfort to your child when everything else appears strange. Around town, it is possible to nurse in subways, buses, in restaurants, parks, or meeting places. Breast-fed babies are excellent travelers.

WHAT IF. . .I want to lose weight while nursing?

After eating well during pregnancy, you should anticipate having ten pounds or so of fat stored on your body for nursing. Usually this fat reserve is used up by the time your baby is six months old. If not, you may safely plan a reducing diet after that time, since your baby will probably start to be interested in solids by this age. Lactation burns about 500 to 1,000 calories a day all by itself, but you don't have to eat a great deal of extra food if you have stored fat from pregnancy. Drinking fluids when thirsty helps to insure a good milk supply. Water, milk, and real juices are the best, most-nutritious fluids. Coffee, tea, and sodas often contain caffeine which can sometimes stimulate the baby excessively by being secreted in the milk.

RECOMMENDATION:

Think of your pregnancy as an 18-month affair instead of 9 months. Your baby is nourished *in utero* 100 percent by what you eat and the same holds true when you are nursing. A relaxed attitude toward your weight after pregnancy will make nursing a more enjoyable experience for you and your family.

WHAT IF. . .I get a plugged duct while nursing?

The breast has a duct system similar to the branches of a tree. If milk clogs a duct, it cannot function and may cause an infection or an abscess. A plugged duct can usually be detected as a hard spot that may be red or tender. The duct must be unplugged as soon as possible so an infection does not develop. The clog may have resulted from a too-tight bra or baby carrier, nursing the baby in the same position all the time so only some ducts are emptied, or from faulty let-down (the release of milk into the ducts).

RECOMMENDATION:

Nurse in varied positions at least every two hours. Apply warm compresses or stand in the shower under a warm spray. Rest between feedings and drink plenty of fluids. If your baby isn't interested in nursing that often, express the milk by hand.

WHAT IF. . .I get a breast infection?

A breast infection feels like the flu. Even if you have no external signs of an infection, only the feeling of malaise that signals flu, assume that you have a breast infection. Follow the recommendations for a plugged duct, but stay in bed. If you have a fever, aspirin may be taken since it passes through the milk in such small quantities that its effects on the baby are negligible.

Antibiotics are frequently prescribed, but research has shown that the primary cure is keeping the breast as empty as possible so the infection cannot fester. If nursing is too painful, milk should be expressed manually or with the aid of a breast pump (the Egnell pump is highly recommended). A doctor who knows the lactating breast should examine the mother for possible abscess. If one has developed, it needs to be drained surgically. None of these things mean that you must terminate nursing. If you have stored milk in your freezer, you can feed the baby your milk from a bottle for a few days until your incision is healed. Better yet, continue to nurse on the unaffected breast. When the incision is healed, resume offering both breasts to your baby.

RECOMMENDATION:

Repeated breast infections may indicate that your diet is not up to par for nursing. You need plenty of vitamin A, a fat-soluble vitamin, to prevent infection and keep your skin in good condition. In general, follow the same basic diet you used for pregnancy when you are nursing to insure that your chances for infection are minimized.

WHAT IF. . .I am dissatisfied with my pediatrician?

Many women choose their children's doctor on the advice of their obstetrician or just because she/he happens to have an office nearby. It is very important to have a good line of communication with your baby's doctor since it will be quite a while before your child will be able to have the primary relationship with the doctor. You should interview them two months or so before your baby is due to find out their attitudes and practices.

RECOMMENDATION:

Ask questions about any aspect of newborn care that puzzles you. Usually, the pediatrician will see the baby only once in the hospital and then not again until the child is one month old.

I was also introduced to the La Leche League through the Bradley classes. This turned out to be very important when I developed a series of minor breast infections in the early weeks of nursing, and the League leader was always ready to give me support and advice about what to do next in order to keep breast feeding. My son is two years old now, and he still likes to nurse a few times each day. It has been a very satisfying experience for me, because I tried to nurse the first baby, but had no information or help in doing so and weaned him at about three weeks. I didn't even try with the next two.

Finding a pediatrician who was supportive of breastfeeding was very traumatic. Our general practitioner said he was supportive when I quizzed him before our baby was born. However, on the second visit with the child, he wanted to introduce solids and said that breast milk was mostly fat and not nutritious.

The pediatrician I have now supports breastfeeding up to 5 or 6 months and has been gently pressuring me to wean my son even though he's thriving on breast milk. I have ignored her and am following the baby's lead, which has meant introducing solids every other day at 5½ months and gradually increasing them so that now, 3 months later, he has three solid meals a day with breast milk when he gets up in the morning, when he goes to bed at night, and between meals. The La Leche League was supportive of my feelings in this matter, too, which helped tremendously.

My search should probably have included finding the right pediatrician. We chose the one who examined the baby after she was born. He supported breast-feeding, but not, it seemed, inquiring parents. Later, when she developed the single problem of her infancy (the lips of her vagina began to adhere), I called and explained the problem to him. He recommended an ointment. In response to my question, he told me it contained a hormone. But reading the package insert which I requested from the druggist, I found the hormone was estrogen, and it appeared to have questionable side effects. I called him again, anxious about using the cream. He became brusque, seemed quite annoyed, and hung up on me, though I had remained courteous to him! I spent the day in tears, feeling helpless. We switched doctors. The group we are with now seems to be more willing to talk over treatments with us.

My mother had a heart attack when our baby was four months old. We spent a bad and busy month helping her cope—in the hospital and at home. Later, I realized that the baby was fussier during that time and didn't gain weight as well. Whether it was my let-down impulse or my rushed behavior, I don't know. Still, I'm glad I didn't do as a local pediatrician advised—start feeding her solids. We weathered the storm. Weaning her then would have deprived me of the solace I felt when she nursed.

Some specific questions to ask:

- What percentage of the babies in your practice are breast-fed for six months or more? (The higher the percentage, the better.)
- When do you suggest solid food be started in the healthy full-term baby? (Around the middle of the first year is the recommended time for the breast-fed baby.)
- Do you make house calls? (If your baby is very sick, it may be important to have a doctor who will come to your house.)
- Who covers for you when you are away? (You may wish to interview this physician also, so you know with whom you will be dealing in case of an emergency.)
- Does the hospital where you have privileges encourage a parent to stay with the child during hospitalization? (The younger the child, the more important it is that a parent be permitted to sleep in during an illness or operation.)
- What are your fees? (Some doctors have a set fee for an entire year of well-baby care; others charge by the visit. Inquire whether any insurance policies you have cover all or part of these costs.)
- If there are dietary, allergic, or other medical problems in your family, you may wish to discuss them with the pediatrician, too.

Another choice for well-baby care might be a nurse-practitioner who works in a clinic or group practice. With clinic care you usually don't get a choice of personnel at each visit. You take whoever is on duty the day of your child's appointment. This alternative may be far less expensive than a private pediatrician, by the way, for well-baby checkups and routine immunizations.

WHAT IF. . .my baby isn't gaining weight?

An infant normally regains his or her birth weight after one week when feeding is done on demand. If this does not happen, the mother needs to evaluate when and how the baby is nursing. Is the baby feeding at least every two or three hours and emptying the breasts at each sitting? Can you feel a rush of milk or a tingling sensation in your nipples or throughout the breast at the beginning of a feeding followed by a general feeling of relaxation? Does the baby suck well? Does the baby spit up a good deal of milk after nursing? Have you introduced a pacifier to the baby? Are you sure your diet is adequate for nursing, so that your milk is of high quality?

RECOMMENDATION:

Try to set up a relaxation time just a minute or two before picking up the baby to nurse. Many women find that sitting down with a beverage and putting their feet up helps them with establishing a let-down reflex. Lying down on your side, your back and head propped with pillows, with the baby nestled next to you is the most relaxing way to nurse. Often, mother and baby drift off to sleep, or, at the very least, enjoy a peaceful interlude in a busy day. You will have trouble nursing in this position if you try to support the baby with your arm. Instead, place the baby on her side directly on the mattress, then position yourself so your breast rests next to her mouth, so she can grasp it easily.

Pacifiers used in combination with nursing can promote or hinder breastfeeding, depending on how they are used. A pacifier is usually a substitute for the mother's nipple, but it cannot duplicate the skin-to-skin contact that is unique to nursing. Too much reliance on the pacifier can dull the baby's appetite or allow the baby to spend a great deal of energy on the sucker. Either way, the baby comes to the breast disinterested in nursing, resulting in a slowdown or stagnation of weight gain.

Pacifiers can aid the mother who temporarily has an overabundance of milk and a baby who wants to suck, but doesn't want milk. A rubber sucker can help the baby with

Breastfeeding is a super relaxer. About a minute after I put my baby to the breast, I feel a mellow wave wash over me, my back releases into the chair or pillow, and I "fog over." At night, I can easily drift off to sleep at her bedtime unless I keep reminding myself of the rest of the night's duties!

When I felt my nipples getting sensitive in the first two days, we tried to have the baby suck on something else for a few hours (my finger, my husband's finger, a clean, damp cloth, a Nuk nipple) while they rested. My baby had a very strong sucking urge which even now she gratifies by sucking her thumb in between feedings (she's 11 months old, eats everything from the table, and also nurses ten times a day!). It's important to meet the baby's needs for sucking—and sometimes it is appropriate to offer something other than the breast.

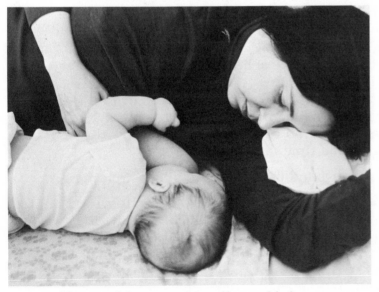

Most restful position for mother and baby.

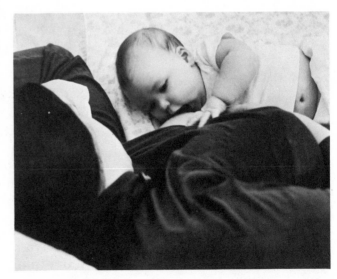

strong sucking needs enjoy life a little more, but should not affect the baby's weight gain.

WHAT IF. . .I get tired easily in the early weeks?

Rest and sleep are vital for the new mother. You must learn to nap and take advantage of whatever rest periods you have during the day. If your childbirth classes featured relaxation techniques, you can use them now to allow your body to rest even if you can't actually sleep during the day.

RECOMMENDATION:

When you come home from the hospital, hopefully after just an overnight stay, plan to spend the first week mostly in bed. Have your husband or helping friend shoo away all those visitors and play with your other children during your naptimes.

Keep the baby in bed next to you so you don't have to get up and go to another room when the baby calls for you. Start by taking three naps a day and cut down only when you feel adequately rested. It is always helpful to have meals frozen in advance so the first week or so after the baby comes you can forget about meal preparation.

Energy is important for motherhood. It takes both physical and emotional strength to take care of an infant. Find all the ways you can to conserve your power. In other cultures, the mother is mothered while she is nursing. This can be your biggest help in the early weeks. Perhaps you could arrange to switch helping weeks with a friend who is also pregnant. Even a kindly cleaning lady can serve this purpose since the tasks that need to be done revolve around housekeeping, not baby care.

Don't make the mistake of hiring a special nurse for the baby. The baby needs interaction with you in the early weeks. Of course, if you have other children, even a high school girl coming in to take them to the park in the afternoon can relieve you of an hour or two of work—and maybe even give you time to take a shower!

WHAT IF. . .my husband feels left out while I'm nursing?

A man doesn't have an active role in breastfeeding per se, but his attitudes have a great deal to do with how successful the mother is at nursing. The father protects the nursing duo from whatever external threats it may encounter (such as critics). Many new fathers report feeling a swell of pride when they see their infant growing so beautifully as the result of exclusive breastfeeding.

RECOMMENDATION:

Each parent has a special role in caring for the infant. Active paternal participation in child care is a relatively new concept. As the nuclear family emerged and men experienced more leisure time, they have been available to their children in more direct ways. Since the baby is an almost completely dependent being, most mothers feel a need to share the responsibility for care with someone. A baby needs far more than simple nourishment. She/he needs love and attention and caressing from both parents. When fathers participate in pregnancy by attending classes and are present at the birth of the child, family bonds are developed. These experiences give the father a special relationship with the newborn.

It was so important for us to have shared this experience. We were both high for days!

While mothers have breasts and milk to give the baby, fathers have strong shoulders for carrying the baby about. A man's wide chest is one of the nicest places for a baby to sleep. And taking baby out for a stroll in the carriage can give mother a needed break toward the end of the day.

WHAT IF. . .I have to return to work?

Virtually all mothers work. Some forms of working are more compatible with nursing than others. Employment outside the home requires some planning, but does not have to mean the end of nursing. A good basic approach to the problem is to remember that some breastfeeding is superior to no breastfeeding.

RECOMMENDATION:

Try to postpone returning to work for at least six to eight weeks after the baby's birth. By this time, you will have an established let-down and you will have had time to become expert at hand expression. Learning how to express milk is important so that when you are separated from your baby, she/he can have your milk and you can be comfortable.

The technique is simple, once you get the knack. The first thing in the morning, after feeding your baby, stroke down the breast from the rib cage and collarbone to the nipple. Rub the areola toward the nipple, then pull the nipple out several times. Put thumb and forefinger above and below the nipple and squeeze them together. After a minute or so, milk will start to come out in drips, then in a fine spray. Expect to express an ounce or two each time. Practice every morning until you can do it with ease. A tea cup or juice glass can be placed underneath the breast to receive the milk if you wish to save it for future use. Breast milk can be frozen (just put it in little freezer bags) and heated later to be served to your baby when you are away.

Finding the right person to care for your baby in your absence is very important. The caretaker should be someone who respects what you are doing. The caretaker's feelings will carry over in the way she treats your baby. Arrange to have the sitter overlap a half hour at the end of the day so you don't have to immediately assume responsi-

HAND EXPRESSION

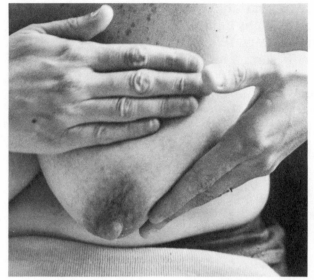
Stroke breast to stimulate milk flow.

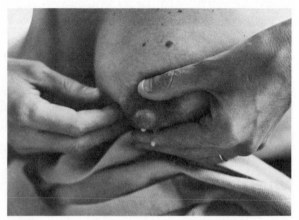
Squeeze areola to start flow.

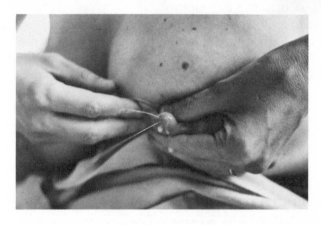
Collect spray of milk for later use.

The La Leche League provides the nursing mother with support at every turn. The women involved at La Leche provided me with a foundation of information at meetings and a network of women to call upon for support and advice. I found all of this extremely valuable and don't expect nursing could have been as rewarding and smooth an experience without their support.

bility for everything when you get home. Instead, you can lie down to nurse the baby while the caretaker puts dinner on or amuses your other children. Don't expect to have all your household chores done, either. Emphasize to the person that taking care of the baby's needs is what is most important to you.

WHAT IF. . .I need consultation about a specific problem or situation?

Call your local La Leche League Leader. She can put you in touch with resource people who can handle almost any problem related to breastfeeding. The national office in Franklin Park, Illinois, also maintains a 24-hour counseling service. All L.L.L.I. assistance is free of charge.

WHAT IF. . .my baby seems to want table food. When should weaning take place?

Weaning begins when your baby starts taking in anything but breast milk. This includes water, juice, crackers, mashed fruits, or supplemental/substitute bottles of formula. When he/she is ready, your baby will indicate an interest in foods the family eats. There is no need for prepared baby foods, by the way. The baby will continue to receive a great deal of nutrition from breast milk for several months after she/he starts picking up small bits of food from a tray and putting them in the mouth. Weaning is a very gradual process that is initiated by the baby and progresses according to the baby's skills at self-feeding.

Make sure that the new foods the baby adds to his/her diet are of high quality. Sweets are not necessary. Nor are special baby juices or prepared meals. Table food, cut into small pieces or mashed with a fork, is far superior to commercially concocted products which have lost much of their nutritional value. An excellent paperback book which outlines sound child nutrition practices and gives specifics for snacks and introducing new foods to your breast-fed baby's diet is:

The Natural Baby Food Cookbook
by Phyllis Williams, R.N., and Margaret Kenda
(New York: Avon Books, 1973)

Even when your child is eating three meals a day with the family, she/he may still want to nurse before a nap or bedtime. This represents an emotional need of your child that should be met long after the time when breastfeeding is critically important from a nutritional point of view. Many children continue this pattern well into the third or fourth year of life, just as those reared on the bottle carry it around with them or latch onto a security object of some sort. You may find that nursing will become more frequent in a toddler or older child who becomes ill. This can prevent dehydration in a child with diarrhea, for instance, thus preventing hospitalization in some cases. Even when the illness is not severe, the gratification that comes from being close to mother is a distinct help to the sick child. Of course, the nutrition provided from your milk is also of great benefit to the child who feels too sick to eat regular meals.

One day, your child will decide she/he doesn't want to nurse anymore. She/he may be playing with siblings and fall asleep before you come in to say good night, or a new baby may arrive and the older child suddenly looks on nursing as something the baby does! However it happens, the end of the nursing relationship is a sign that you have met your child's needs in a way that only *you* could accomplish. It should set the tone for your continuing relationship with your child, a loving give-and-take that is mutually satisfying for both people.

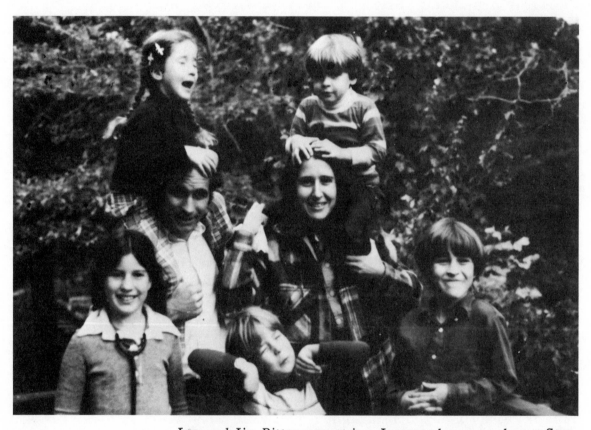

Jane and Jim Pittenger met in a Japanese language class at Stanford University. She was a peace marcher; he marched in ROTC.

Today they live in North Haven, Connecticut with Bede, 13; Niguelle, 10; Sol, 8; Jasmine, 6; and Basil, 4. Jane is a graduate student in Yale University's School of Nursing Maternal-Newborn Program which leads to a certificate in Nurse-Midwifery. Jim is a marriage and family counselor and full-time father while Jane is busy in school.

Over the past ten years, the Pittengers have been active in childbirth education, lactation counseling, and parent education. They are now affiliated with the Parent Effectiveness Training and Counseling Service and FAMILY, Family-Centered Childbirth and Parenting, a group which trains and supports couple-teachers of childbirth education. They have coauthored several articles on childbearing and its effects on marriage and family relations.

6

Pregnancy Means Parenting

by: Jane G. Pittenger
and James E. Pittenger

Supplied as we are with dazzling photographs of fetal development, it is relatively easy for any interested person to understand the importance of the nine months of pregnancy for babies. At no other time in their lives are they so totally vulnerable and dependent on their parents as during this period. It is harder to realize how important pregnancy is to the adults who must turn into parents during this time. The very real acts of parenting performed or not performed during pregnancy have lasting effects on both parent and child. By consciously caring for the baby before she/he is born, parents can develop to their fullest potential the opportunities pregnancy provides for personal enrichment and growth.

However, like their baby, budding parents are at risk during pregnancy, too. Unless they acknowledge the need for active parenting, they might restrict the development of their child and themselves, with negative results that are both immediate and long lasting. Yet expectant parents in our society receive little help in recognizing pregnancy as a richly rewarding time in its own right, rather than merely a long wait for the big event.

In many ways, though we have a fascination with birth itself, it would appear that pregnancy is totally unnoticed by most Americans, neatly ignored except as a medical matter presided over by doctors. Pregnant women receive little attention as thinking and feeling individuals. Even those doctors with more humanistic tendencies tend to reduce pregnancy to

> an interaction among four important Ps—a woman's parity (the number of previous births she has had), the pelvis, the perineum (the tissue around the vagina), and her psychology.

—Howard Berk, M.D., in the Foreword to *Pregnancy After 35* by C.S. McCauley (New York: Dutton, 1976)

How do parents react to their own pregnancy in the face of this cultural "blacklisting"? In trying to answer this question in a 1977 article in *Keeping Abreast Journal* (vol. II, no. 1. "Perinatal Period: Breeding Ground for Marital or Parental Maladjustment"), we wrote:

> The present cultural view of pregnancy is that it is . . . a

How well I remember parenting Elise while she was still within me. I'd lie in bed and feel her movements, and I'd respond to them by caressing my belly and murmuring love sounds to her. Frequently, I'd talk to her, telling her how happy she made me and how I longed to gather her up and cuddle her in my arms. I was constantly sending out love vibrations.

The most important thing for me was making pregnancy and childbirth a joint venture with Jim. I needed this psychologically. I was not going to go through it alone!

My psychological preparation and well-being during pregnancy were indeed strengthened by Jim's understanding and support. It wasn't always easy for him, because of my physical discomforts and feelings of loneliness which even he couldn't alleviate, but he empathized with me as best he could.

165

joke, an obscenity, or a disease. Most husbands and wives spend many of their pregnant days laughing at it, hiding from it, or acting the role of the long-suffering patient. No one has attempted to measure the consequences of playing Jester, Fugitive, and Martyr . . . on one's subsequent capacities as a parent. . . .

However, parents need not subscribe to the common way of looking at pregnancy. If they seek to make the most of the experience, they will come to see it differently. As Libby and Arthur Colman wrote in *Pregnancy: The Psychological Experience* (New York: The Seabury Press, 1973):

Pregnancy is neither a static nor a brief experience, but one full of growth, change, and enrichment . . . a time when one's life impinges directly on the most basic psychological and physiological processes, when abstractions like fertility, fulfillment, and death become of more immediate and personal concern . . . as rewarding as it is challenging . . . for, at the end, there is literally a new life, for the parents as well as for the child.

Pregnancy Is a Stage of Parenthood

Programs for enriching pregnancy are rare. Traditional childbirth classes focus on labor and birth. Even reading material dealing with pregnancy apart from issues of health is scarce. Parenting classes emphasize the trials and pleasures of living with young babies.

Our approach is to view pregnancy as a stage of parenthood and to encourage parents to assume command of this experience as they would any other vital aspect of their lives. If you are pregnant, you are already parenting. You have earned the title mother or father by your decision to continue this pregnancy. You have already begun to nurture your baby and to undergo changes yourself.

Today there are many options available to you as over-30 parents dealing with decisions during pregnancy. You can place yourself in an extremely favorable position, physically and emotionally, by participating to the maximum in all phases of your pregnancy and birth. You have absolute control over the critical factors which bear most directly on the health of yourself and your baby—nutrition, exercise, education, and selection of medical care. As an older individual, you have had years to develop decision-making skills which you could not have brought to these matters as a younger parent.

We were determined to let no one interfere in what we knew would be a beautiful, healthy childbirth. We were extremely protective of our soon-to-be-born child and would not risk any damage to her whatsoever by any intrusion upon the natural birth process. This was our baby, and it was our responsibility to assure her the safest birth possible.

Still, many parents think the most important task confronting them at the beginning of their pregnancy is to select a medical care provider and leave the responsibility for all these decisions to him/her! The result of this attitude is that the entire outcome of the pregnancy is based on what someone other than the parents decides.

We want to share with you some concepts and activities we have developed to help the parents become active participants in each pregnancy while developing their own approach to parenting. Try to explore each area thoroughly with your partner before going on to the next. One last point: Much of this material is new, and you may well find yourselves refining it as you work through the topics. If you do, please share it with us.

The "Mine!" Concept

Saying "No" and "Mine" is a vital part of human development which we parents need to understand and accept in our children. These assertions are part of the necessary process of becoming an individual, of growing apart from one's parents and facing the challenges of life independently. In short, it is a way of saying, "I am mine; I want a say in how this is handled."

As we begin to become parents we also need to say "Mine" to ourselves, to our child, and to society. It is a basic step in developing our individual characteristics as parents. One important result is that the parent perceives parenting as an integral part of her-/himself, not just a duty, task, or social role. The mother and father become attached to their infant, feel that their infant is immensely important, feel a need to protect and nurture their baby, and find a great measure of self-affirmation in their relationship.

Doctors Marshall Klaus and John Kennel of Case Western Reserve University, well-known researchers of the process of human maternal-infant attachment, have concluded:

> The power of this attachment is so great it enables the mother or father to make the unusual sacrifices necessary for the care of their infant day after day, night after night. . . . This bond is the wellspring for all the infant's subsequent attachments and is the formative relationship in the course of which the child develops a sense of himself.

One prerequisite is a decision to stand apart from others, to make up our own minds about caring for our children in ways that have meaning for us. Parents who choose this approach to child rearing should be prepared for

While I was pregnant, I continued to do everything I did before. In fact, I did more: I never missed a class or a day at work. I felt I had to prove that being pregnant was just like not being pregnant.

The hospital policy for rooming-in at the time I had my baby included a 24-hour interim between delivery and rooming-in. Of course I fought with the hospital. I felt like a toddler saying, "Mine, mine, mine."

We decided we wanted to be together for this baby's birth, and because we were older and less worried about making a fuss, I started asking the doctor in the clinic to get permission for my husband to come into the labor and delivery rooms with me. We knew the hospital had made a few exceptions to its rules in recent years; so we were determined to do it our way. Our Bradley childbirth teacher was very helpful, always stressing to us how we could deal effectively with whatever circumstances came up. We received a card at the end of the series which stated that my husband was a trained labor and birth coach. He kept it in his wallet, and it turned out to be an important piece of paper.

On the day our baby was born, the doctor I had seen in the clinic was out of the hospital. Luckily, I arrived there late in labor and was taken directly to the delivery room. But my husband was barred from entering the delivery area by the resident who was going to do the delivery. My husband could hear me calling for him to come in, and he was getting frantic with the resident who barely spoke English and who finally threw up his hands and took my husband into the office of the OB/GYN chief who just happened to be in his office.

My husband told him that the clinic doctor had okayed it for him to be with me; he pulled out his coach card and said he'd been trained to help during the birth, and he threatened to sue the hospital if he weren't allowed in! The OB/GYN chief just looked at him, shook his head, and told the resident to let him in. By this time, the baby was almost out, and we were together for the last push.

society to react in a way not much different from the way an angry parent reacts to a naughty toddler.

It may start with the obstetrician who berates a couple who want to leave the hospital with their new baby a few hours after birth if all goes well. Then comes the nursing supervisor who refuses to deviate from hospital routine no matter what the needs of individual parents and babies. And don't forget the guys at work who hassle a man who wants to be with his wife during labor and birth. All seem to be threatened in some way by the parents' efforts to control the course of pregnancy and childbirth.

Some Encourage a Take-Charge Attitude among Parents

A small segment of the medical establishment, aware of the conclusions reached by researchers like Klaus and Kennel, is beginning to encourage this take-charge attitude among parents, instead of opposing it. Some hospitals are gradually removing restrictions on early, intimate contact between parents and infants. Progressive institutions are abandoning such practices as routine medication of the mother for labor and birth, forced separation of parents and infants at birth, feeding by schedule, ignoring or discouraging breastfeeding, wrapping babies so that touching is interfered with, and keeping babies segregated in a central nursery rather than being cared for at the mothers' bedsides. Optionally, parents are urged to assume responsibility for their babies to the extent they desire and develop competence in meeting their babies' needs before leaving the hospital.

Encouraging parental self-assertion has a long way to go, though. It runs counter to strong cultural currents. Most parents encounter and have to deal with a pattern of professional concern for parenting that typically intervenes by way of "advice":

Doctor Spock's *Baby and Child Care* says I should. . . .
Doctor Rutherford's *You and Your Baby* says she should . . . .
Doctor Brazelton's *Infants and Mothers* says he should . . . .
Doctor White's *The First Three Years of Life* tells us not to . . . .

Such edicts are pitfalls to new parents or those trying to modify their parenting style, because they give the impression that there is a correct way to dealing with every aspect of parenting. The issue is not whether the advice given is good. Its detrimental effect is that parents are taught to look to others, rather than to themselves, for solutions to parenting problems. They learn to be helpless, irresponsible, exploited. Eventually, because neither they nor their children can meet the expectations implied by the advice-givers, they finally give up on parenting. In effect, they say, "Let someone else (the school, the church, the social workers, the psychiatrist, the neighbors, the grandparents) raise my children. I give up!"

Variation among human individuals is enormous. It follows that relationships between parents and children will not lend themselves to prescribed rules for behavior. Because each relationship is a dynamic, changing give-and-take, it is unrealistic to hope that anyone not involved closely with it can understand and help the partners fulfill themselves in it.

A final obstacle to parental individuation lies not with society as a whole, but within ourselves. Most of us hesitate, at one stage or another, as we assume full responsibility for a child. Parents simultaneously welcome and resist the changes which are inevitable as one becomes a parent: less personal freedom, less insulation from intimate contact with others, and more hard work. Parents show their ambivalence about these changes and their imperatives for investigating and relying on their own resources in many ways. For example, expectant couples may openly fret about their doctor through an entire series of childbirth classes, yet never quite give in to their negative feelings about him or her and switch to another.

In counseling, our main effort is directed toward freeing parents from the "shoulds" and "oughts" of society, old and new, and encouraging them to rely on their own genuine feelings and good sense. Though it requires a big effort, the ability to say "Mine" is a fundamental step in becoming a parent.

To explore where you are in the process of self-assertion, try this activity, developed with the help of Elaine Small of Lynbrook, New York, a fellow Parent Effectiveness Training Instructor.

We found, as parents who had never had a child before—or even known what a baby was like, that Dr. Spock's Baby and Child Care and Burton White's The First Three Years were reassuring, especially during the particularly scary first three months. Basically, both books told us that everything was normal. What they didn't cover, our local La Leche leader helped us with.

It meant a great deal to me to be able to walk around, eat lightly, and enjoy the peace and warmth of my own home and bed. It is really the way every baby should be welcomed into the world. Probably the most wonderful part of having him at home was that my husband and I were never separated from the baby. I took him directly into bed with me where we got to know him right away. We all just snuggled together in an unbelievably warm, wonderful way. The love and bonding that flowed between us seemed so extremely right and so extremely the opposite of the cold rigidity of hospital births.

Set Up Your Own Pregnancy, Inc. Board of Directors

Draw a diagram of a board of directors (see below). Then think about your pregnancy and the people, living and dead, who are helping you make decisions about it. Place their names by each chair. Add or subtract chairs as you wish.

The following example was provided by a first-time father, age 34, whose wife was eight months pregnant at the time.

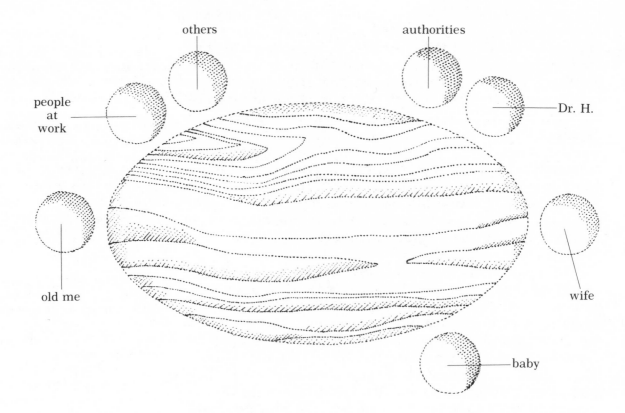

In analyzing your Pregnancy, Inc. Board of Directors, try to decide who is included and where they are sitting in relation to you and each other. Who is doing most of the talking? To whom? Who would you like to hear more of? Less of? What strengths and weaknesses do you see?

This man observed that his wife was really the person in charge of his experience with pregnancy. He was bound to her far more than to their baby, and his own participation stemmed from her decisions and needs. His main interest was in her as his partner; he had little conscious reaction to being a father.

This disinterest troubled him, and he postulated a "New Me" which might emerge from the experiences of pregnancy and birth in which he was taking an active part. This "New Me" would presumably feel more fatherly than the "Old Me" seated at the far end of the table. He felt that most of the individuals involved with pregnancy—Doctor H., the natural childbirth authorities, and baby—were closer to his wife than to him. He felt left out of her experiences and slightly envious of her. But he did not feel abandoned by her; in fact, her interest in his reactions, enthusiastic appreciation of pregnancy, and desire to have him share in birth and parenting said quite the opposite, that she needed his full attention now more than before. Sometimes he felt

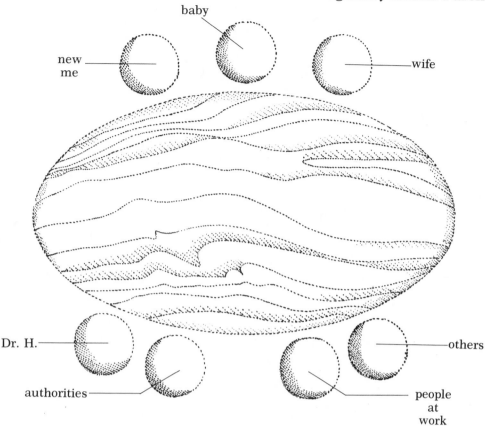

an urge to find projects of his own; to escape the intensity and monotony of her interests. Also, he was surprised at her new sexual aggressiveness, although not dismayed by it.

As he evaluated his Board of Directors, he came to appreciate himself more and drew his "New Me" chair larger. A conflict existed between his new and old selves to be sure, but he was taking an active part in dealings with Doctor H., reading and practicing for birth, and trying to work up an interest in the baby *in utero*. He could see changes in himself over the past months of pregnancy that indicated a growing involvement in this new facet of his marriage, and he could see that he was, in terms of action, becoming more of a father all the time.

On the other hand, he was disturbed about some of the weaknesses he saw. His lack of feeling about the baby was one of these. Another was the absence of friends (perhaps men like himself) who would share his ambivalence, understand it, yet encourage him in his quest toward full fatherhood. He wished he were closer to his own father and father-in-law. He wished his fellow employees were more approving of natural childbirth but was grateful that, although they thought him strange, they did not ridicule him. He became aware that he was basically lonely with his wife (his only real friend) absorbed in pregnancy. He realized that he was frightened that the baby, when it came, would mean the loss of his only companion.

In brief, he saw strengths in his "New Me," in his relationship with his wife, and in their ability to place Doctor H., natural childbirth authorities, and the expected baby in a more or less subordinate position to their marriage. He decided that he had made some progress toward becoming a father and that now he needed to take a closer look at his fear of being left alone, his lack of friends, and his blah feelings about the baby, to see what he could do about them.

The Perfect Child Concept

In a recent article parents were asked, "Why did you decide to have a child?" One father replied that he was not quite sure but that he thought it would be nice to teach his child how to make the world a better place. One of the psychologists asked to contribute her views on the subject stated, "If he has no better reason than that, he is in for trouble!" Unfortunately, she never said what a good reason would be. So we and the other readers still do not know whether we had children for the right reasons or not.

The one thing we are sure of when we ask this question is that most of the parents in the crowd will feel uncomfortable. They are afraid that they did not have the right reason for becoming parents, so they can't hope to be good parents with decent children. This discomfort and fear stem from one of the most persistent and most questionable beliefs we parents have: Parenting is a job, and our children are products.

I think I can look at Rachael more objectively in her development than I would have been able to at 20, letting her be herself and providing the environmental elements necessary for that development. My earlier approach to a child would have been more demanding and precise.

Of course there are drawbacks. We are not planning to have another child. To raise this one unspoiled, to put her in life arenas early enough so that she can experience the give and take of other children, and to be able to respond to a child 40 years younger—these concerns are realities we must face.

The idea of parenting as person production leads to an evaluation of children and parents in terms of stereotypes rather than as individuals. It leads to tremendous anxiety on the part of parents (particularly young parents) and children as they wonder, "Am I an alright mother?" "Am I ruining my children?" "Am I an OK child?" Its most destructive effect, however, is that it discourages parents from evaluating themselves and their children on their own terms instead of someone else's. Parents deny their own uniqueness and that of their children by focusing on ill-defined external standards about what is proper in child and parent.

Who Has a Perfect Formula for Child Rearing?

One gets the impression that someone actually knows how to produce a decent, if not perfect, human being. Writers about child rearing certainly give the impression that the rules for successful parenting have been discovered and carved in stone and, if applied properly, are effective. Dr. Richard Farson, however, maintains otherwise. In a summer, 1976 address to teachers of Parent Effectiveness Training, he described his review of the literature on child rearing practices. A major finding was that no one has demonstrated that any specific approach to child rearing has a significantly greater chance of producing a certain type of child than any other. His analysis, at least casts doubt on the validity of theories of child rearing, and suggests that, for the time being, parents can relax and forget about whether or not theirs is the correct way to raise children.

Dr. Farson encourages parents to view children as people instead of as products. This seems so obvious— children *are* people—that it comes as a shock to discover how unlike people we parents perceive them to be. Many adults consider children another form of life, not quite ready for full human contact.

It is a double-edged sword we wield when we allow ourselves to think this way. We forbid ourselves to share our fears and hurts with our child ("Might be too much for him. . ."). We cannot rely on our feelings in confronting him or her, but must appeal to some higher order that confers special powers upon parents ("Because I'm your mother, that's why!"). We feel obliged to show anger when our true feelings may be something far different. We relate to our children as leaders but seldom as fellow human beings. Even more rarely do we seek them out as individuals who can give us help and comfort when we need it!

The Failure Concept

Sooner or later, we parents find ourselves failing to live up to our own standards. For example, not more than 20 of the more than 150 couples who have taken our family-centered childbirth course reported that they had had a perfect labor and birth, despite a very low rate of medication and a very high rate of positive experiences overall. Feelings of personal failure were much stronger in women whose birth experience fell *short* of their expectations. Speaking of women who intended to have natural childbirth but wound up with Cesarean sections, Dr. Leonard Safon, who is a member of the C/SEC advisory board, remarked; "It's frightening what they think. . . . A lot hated their doctors and a lot of them hated themselves because they failed."

Pregnant parents, of course, suffer from *thoughts* of failure, too. The older ones worry that they waited too long to conceive and that their baby will be defective. At all ages

My attitude toward child raising and mothering has drastically changed in the 15 years between having my first and second child. With the first child, I was more prone to worry about not spoiling the child. I realize now that love never spoils, only causes growth, mutual love, and understanding between child and parent.

I would let my first cry it out at times, but I can't bear to allow crying now with the second baby. I even went to work (under the intimidation of my previous husband) only five weeks after the birth of my first child. I would never do that now with an infant unless my child could be with me on the job. I simply could not and would not tolerate separation at this stage in his life.

One problem during pregnancy was finding out that one of our doctors was not favorable to Lamaze. Both Jim and I made the effort to set up special visits with each doctor to tell each our wishes. Besides having a conservative view toward natural childbirth, the one doctor's main objection stemmed from my age. His experience was that women who are older and who had no previous births do not have the suppleness required for a completely natural delivery. Our Lamaze teacher had encouraged us, of course; so we were positive in our approach, but we were realistic, too. We did discuss the drugs I would and would not want to use with the doctor—in case I needed them.

This visit proved invaluable because the objecting doctor was on duty the evening I went into labor. (He subsequently delivered the baby.) The breathing throughout my 13 hours of labor was most helpful until the last 40 minutes when I could no longer maintain any motor control—the labor contractions lasted 2 to 2½ minutes each with less than 30 seconds in between. (Even Lamaze didn't prepare us for this!) We had decided beforehand, during that visit, that, should difficulties arise, I would ask for a saddle block. This I did.

Although it was a disappointment to me to have to ask for it, the saddle block was necessary. But I was awake during delivery, and I was able to push and be an active participant in Rachael's birth. This surprised the doctor. Jim coached me from the beginning of labor until birth.

they fear that medication and other drugs taken during pregnancy may harm the child. They hope that they have not damaged the baby through frightening dreams, that their diet is nutritious enough, that they have chosen a skilled doctor or midwife, and so on.

It is important to recognize that failure is part of parenting. By failing at times to fulfill our expectations as parents, we gradually come to discover who we are, to know our limitations, our special qualities, our needs and those of our child. But failure is painful; it evokes sorrow and anger, guilt and fear, and ambivalence.

Angela McBride in her book, *The Growth and Development of Mothers* (New York: Harper and Row, 1973), calls these negative feelings that parents frequently experience "normal crazies." Unfortunately, many parents believe that they have failed just by having these "wrong" feelings about parenthood. After all, aren't parents supposed to be always loving, patient, wise, stable, gentle but firm, and sensitive to the needs of children? No parent wants to stray from this ideal. When reality clashes with our expectations of ourselves and our children, we wonder where we went wrong—instead of realizing that this may be a helpful part of the growing process adults undergo as they become parents.

Imagine Your Dream Child

Dr. James Murphy, a New York City psychiatrist with special interest in early parent-infant interaction, uses this exercise in his workshops to assist parents in confronting their tendency to idealize their children and themselves.

Try imagining your dream baby—tender, satiny smooth skin, a curl maybe, cuddlesome, smiley, pink-cheeked, good-natured—and list his or her characteristics on a scrap of paper, trying to be as specific as possible. Then imagine the parent of such a baby—patient, sensitive, playful, creative—and mark these characteristics of the good parent on another piece of paper. Dr. Murphy has parents tape these preconceived ideas of the "good" parent and the "good" baby to the wall for the duration of the workshops, and tells them to try to relate to their babies as people, instead.

In your pregnant state, you can do this also. Post these papers somewhere conspicuous, and note in passing the differences between the real you and the real child inside and the dream persons posted to the wall.

After a day or two of noting the contrast between the baby and parent you hope for and the real versions, take the papers from the wall and burn them. Acknowledge your failure to produce the baby of your dreams and to become the parent of your dreams. Say goodbye. It is possible that you will feel a flicker of anger and loss as you do this. Imagine how much greater this is when, after years of trying, parents finally begin to acknowledge that neither they nor their child has ever borne a close resemblance to the dream.

Learn How to Risk It

Competent risk-taking leads to peace of mind, easier decisions, greater acceptance of disaster in case it happens, more flexibility, more control of events, greater self-respect, and enhanced appreciation of life.

With your partner, try this experiment in coping with risk. Repeat it as fears of new dangers arise during pregnancy.

Discover your fears first; identify what is risky about pregnancy for you. Privately record your fears without any particular order. Include little things as well as big; e.g. a baby with a nose like a potato, a boy when you want a girl, a child handicapped in some way. Afterwards, rank them, placing the risk that most troubles you first. Focus on just those highest-ranked items for the remaining time.

Next, define the risks involved with your partner. Take plenty of time for this, and try to help each other develop a complete picture of where that fear comes from, what it looks like, why it is especially upsetting, what it would be like to live with if it actually materialized, and what you would do about it. Try to avoid reassuring each other, and dismiss the impulse to shrug it off as either unimportant or something one has no control over. What matters is that it is real as a fear. (At another time you may want to define the risks more accurately by investigating real cases where your fear has materialized. If mongolism is on your list, read about it. If possible, work with a mongoloid child. Talk with his parents. Perhaps this risk is not as great as it seems; or perhaps it is greater.)

After sharing, confront your fears. The one who owns the fear relaxes—lying or sitting comfortably—closes her eyes, breathes easily, relaxes muscle groups from head to toes—and when relaxed, signals her partner with a raised fingertip that she is ready. Speaking slowly, her partner describes the fear in degrees, in scenes ranging in intensity from slightly upsetting to moderately upsetting. For instance, seeing a mongoloid child might evoke a mild fear. Caring for a mongoloid child for a half-hour at the park might be more frightening. Being mother to a mongoloid child might be the most distressing scene possible.

Meanwhile, the owner of the fear remains relaxed and pictures the various scenes in her mind. If she feels herself tensing up, the owner should signal her partner to stop. She should then attempt to relax again and resume the activity. End the exercise after two stop signals. It is important to go slowly for this experience to be effective.

Close the exercise by sharing your thoughts and feelings. Then switch places.

Resume the experiment at another time, on a regular basis perhaps, either continuing with the original risk or adding another from your lists.

Finally, do what you can to minimize the danger. Study the subject thoroughly. Look at the benefits as well as the risks of alternatives available to you. Make a written plan. Post it and follow it conscientiously. Ask your partner to help you carry out your plan.

Concentrate on Now

Another way of turning away from parenting is by focusing on the future. While pregnant, we dream of sweet little babies; when the kids are infants, we cannot wait until they learn to walk; when toddlers, the goal is nursery school; when 6 to 10, we hope they will soon be able to do their share of the housework and take care of themselves; when preteens and teens, we anticipate the day they move out; and then, we anxiously await grandchildren. Each stage of parenthood has its problems, to be sure, but coping by looking to the future for solutions is escape. The irony of it is that we can escape the positive features of parenthood: intimacy, play, touching and holding, the beauty of young bodies, sharing, and growth, but we cannot escape most of the annoyances: the noise, chaos, slow pace, bills, unpredictability, responsibility of thinking for others, disruptions of home and lifestyle, interference with career, and so forth. Using escape to improve the parenting experience accents the negative and mutes the positive.

If it is difficult for many parents to live in the present during infancy, toddlerhood, and so on, it is even harder during pregnancy. According to our cultural myth, pregnancy *is* looking to the future. It is given no significance other than as a medical and biological event. It is also unpleasant, being jampacked with the likes of nausea, dizziness, hemorrhoids, and frightening dreams. Popular wisdom has it that the mature woman toughs her way through all this. She puts parenting off, limits her involvement, diminishes her parental self.

I had put off having a child to what I considered the last moment, considering the rising risks of fetal abnormalities and my age. I had a career and was accustomed to being independent, active, and physically strong. My confidence and sense of well-being were built upon looking well, doing what I wanted, and upon my relationship with my husband. Being pregnant changed all that. I felt grossly fat. I had a rash on my face for the first time (even as a teenager I'd had clear skin). My movements were lumbering and slow. I couldn't understand how anyone could love me. I couldn't do things with my usual efficiency toward the end of my pregnancy, nor could I think with my usual clearness. It was not the high point in my life.

I would have been an awful parent at age 25. I was much too interested in myself and my career to pay attention to a child. I would have resented the time a baby takes.

It was incumbent upon me to prove that the condition of my pregnancy did not in any way interfere with my work. My heroines were women I had heard of who worked 18-hour days until the onset of labor and returned a week later as if nothing more than a toothache had been responsible for their absence. The only good pregnant woman was one who kept her morning sickness and hemorrhoids to herself. And so, I rarely publicized and barely even acknowledged the child to come. When pressed, I would shrug it off: "Who, me? Pregnant?"

Against this background, it is a wonder that we still hear remarks like, "Oh, I loved being pregnant. I felt like a walking miracle!" Or, as Libby Colman writes in *Pregnancy: the Psychological Experience* (New York: The Seabury Press, 1973):

> The excitement of carrying an invisible baby in the first trimester is as intense and romantic as falling in love. It brings on the same spurts of joy, the same intense desire to sing and skip down the street, the same feeling of being more special than anybody else in the world. If that happiness starts to fade, it is renewed by the baby's first movements, for now the woman has a chance to fall in love with her state all over again.
>
> Finally, in the ninth month, a woman reaches one of the most beatific phases of human existence. She acquires a physical form which has stimulated not only art but worship throughout the ages.

Here is what happened when one mother stopped running and instead plunged into the choppy waters of parenting:

> Many I know of similar age to me look at me and my baby and say either to themselves or to me openly, "Better you than me." I have also been in that place. It is almost impossible to tell them in words what having my late-in-life baby has done for me and what she gives to me on a daily basis. My baby helps me to rediscover the wonder of a starlit sky, the sound of rain, the brilliance and fragrance of a simple, stray, wild flower. I love to watch her explore, to observe her discovery of how one little finger can pry loose a piece of bark on a giant spruce tree, to see her enjoy the feel of mud between her toes and the sensation of water from the hose, icy cold from our well deep in the ground. Bugs and birds, the rhythm of music, the good feeling of moving one's body, the sourness of a lemon, the sweetness of honey, her mastery of new skills—all these things and more bring her pleasure. I love to hear her say, "I did it myself," and "I very angry." Basic truths, basic beauties—daily I learn the lessons life has for us: joy and pain, the bittersweet mixture all fresh, all new through my baby. What more could I need or want or ask for? My life is so good, so full; she gives me so much to grow on. Together we share, together we love, is

The doctor said, "One more push and you'll have your baby." I debated for a moment—do I want to push and have a baby; or do I want to get up, walk out, and continue being pregnant.

How proud I was with this pregnancy. I had returned to school at the time, and there I was, among all those young college girls, blossoming forth in all my glory, the center of attraction and endless questions. I relished every moment of it.

Because childbearing and birth are such an integral part of one's being, I tend to think that it was better for me to experience them as a woman of 40 than as a woman in my 20s. Although I was not ready psychologically at the precise time of the discovery that I was pregnant, I was ready in the broader sense as I look over my entire life picture.

I am a calmer, more relaxed woman now than I was at 20; I am more interested in the essentials of a full life than in the trappings and perfectionist views of my youth. My life experiences have been wholesome and conducive to growth. My Christian beliefs and values have given me an appreciation for human life and freedom, with my years of teaching and counseling only enhancing this appreciation.

there anything in this world more important? Is there?

(Sarah's baby, Suzy, is about two years old. You have heard of the Terrible Twos?)

The temptation to dismiss these women as incurable romantics is strong. It may seem as if they were looking for miracles, exaggerating brief bubbles of emotion, seizing on feelings and fantasies beyond reason. But it may be otherwise. It may be that they spent less time running from their pregnant selves and more time making acquaintances.

The Concept of Self-Awareness and Self-Interest

It takes some courage just to mention self-interest in the same sentence with parenting in the face of beliefs that parenthood is selfless, giving, concerned above all for the child's future, and preoccupied with providing the "right" upbringing. But without attending to their own needs, parents sabotage their efforts to do well by their children.

Since contraception and abortion have become available, more people who become parents chose to do so. They want to love their children and be loved in turn. But this commitment to the high ideals of love does not prepare them for actually loving—the give and take of love—on a daily basis.

I had my first child at age 18, the second at age 33. Concerning my second, I thought I had passed the age physically—but mostly, emotionally—for further childbearing. I felt I had all the patience in the world at age 18, but I now find this is not so—just the opposite is true! At 18 I was still growing up, but now I have exceedingly greater patience; also a much more maternal attitude. I am sure this has much to do with the naturalness and ease of my home birth and nursing this baby.

I also feel that the children of younger women are less appreciated, less cherished, and, in some ways, neglected or "shoved off" on other people. My second child I view as a gift, whereas my first seemed more of a responsibility.

There are times when I am not in a giving posture, when I need time and space to me for me. I now know that is OK! Not only OK, but essential for my own personal survival. I am more in touch with me—my feelings, my needs—and have begun to realize how to express them, how to openly declare them. This whole process makes giving to others easier. When feelings, whether on a conscious or subconscious level, go unrecognized or are not expressed, they don't go away. They submerge, simmer, smoulder, and change to resentment, and resentment makes *free* giving impossible. These are the things I did not know or understand at age 23, 25, 28, or even 33; now at age 39 I do, and did when my fifth baby was born at 38.

I am continuing to grow. I have an increasing sense of who I am for me. The more I am, the more I become, and the more I have to give to my baby and the freer I am to give it. Being freer to give, I am freer to receive. It is truly beautiful to begin having a love affair with life, my husband, my baby, at the age of 40.

Awareness—that's the key. That's what I have gained as I have grown and matured!

Too often, parents do not know themselves well enough to know what they can give. They feel they should give as parents, regardless of whether giving suits their personal needs or not. They give time when they have not enough for themselves; they take their children to the playground when perhaps they need to play, too. Even when these parents deny their children, it is usually not because they personally object to the giving but because they feel that they should refuse those things for the child's good.

Inappropriate giving results in feelings of resentment and unhappiness in the parent. She feels hurt and tends to withdraw from the relationship. Less of the parent remains involved in the relationship with the child each time this withdrawal occurs, and parenting takes on a sour note. A negative cycle is established, with guilt ("I ought to give") inducing the parent to give inappropriately (lack of self-awareness), leading to hurt and anger and then withdrawal by the parent. The parent senses that her withdrawal contradicts her belief in selfless giving, feels even more guilty, and is inclined to continue the cycle through more inappropriate giving.

With greater self-awareness and self-interest, parents can reduce the unrealistic demands they make on themselves for giving, recognize that feelings of resentment and unhappiness are in large part their own doing, and counteract the inclination to escape through withdrawing from their children. Also, with self-awareness comes a sense of self-expansion: There seems to be much more of one's self available for giving, and sharing seems easier. Awareness also leads to increased appreciation for the gifts the child has to offer. A positive cycle of giving and receiving develops, generating greater parent-child bonding, quite the opposite of the guilt-hurt-anger-withdrawal cycle.

Indulge Yourself With Twenty Likes

Child rearing and baby carrying are usually less burdensome than we allow them to be. We need to watch ourselves carefully. Are our needs as individuals being met? Are we falling into unawareness and unintentional martyrdom?

Try this exercise adapted from Sidney B. Simon's *Values Clarification* (New York: Hart Publishing Co., 1972) for a reading on where you stand in relationship to pregnancy. Draw a grid like the one below with 20 rows and 11 columns. Fill in the columns one at a time starting at the left and moving to the right, according to the directions at the head of each column.

The example given was done by Rachel, a mother with a toddler, but the principle remains the same throughout parenting, pregnancy included.

There was a drastic change in my relationship to my husband and in our lifestyles that was confusing and upsetting, because we didn't expect it. We were used to doing what we pleased and were completely absorbed in each other. After the baby arrived, I was completely absorbed in it and in my recovery. I didn't understand why my husband was jealous of the child and didn't share my overwhelming concern for the baby. The child is becoming more independent now, and we're adjusting with difficulty. I am freer to give my husband more time, and he realizes that we can't have the relationship we had before the baby was born and that he must share in the care of the child. If we'd known about these difficulties before the child was born, it wouldn't have been so hard.

I List 20 things you like to do	II If you do it alone, mark A; with others, P; both, AP	III If some risk, mark R	IV If it costs more than $3.00, mark $	V If it was not on your list five years ago, mark –	VI If you want to do more of it in the five years to come, mark +
Swim	AP	R			+
Make love	AP	R			+
Dream about baby	A			–	+
Do relaxation (with coach)	AP			–	+
Get high	AP	R	$		+
Rock climbing	AP	R			+

VII	VIII	IX	X	XI
Does pregnancy interfere with it?	Will having an infant interfere?	What date did you do it last?	Rank order your 10 favorites #1, #2, #3, etc.	Contract with self
Encourage = E Prohibit = PR Restrict = RES No Change = N				
E	RES	9/76	4	I will arrange to swim several times a week.
E	PR RES	Yesterday	2	I will talk to Sam about ways of making love without intercourse when baby is born.
E	Actualize dreams	Today	5	I will stop feeling guilty about "wasting" time dreaming about my baby.
E	RES	A week ago	8	I will make a deal with Sam and a friend to do relaxation after baby is born.
PR	PR RES	9/76	10	I will talk to Sam and a friend about my need to stay sober with a baby inside and outside. Will try to avoid feeling left out, maybe find no-drug ways of getting high.
RES	PR RES	10/76	7	I will get a "holder-sitter" for the baby and take her with us two months after birth. For now, I will plan two climbs for after the birth.

What This List Reveals

Rachel likes to do her favorite things with someone, usually Sam. Most of the things she likes also involve some degree of risk, whether it be personal exposure as in lovemaking, or physical danger as in rock climbing. Cost does not appear to be a handicap, for most of her pleasures are inexpensive. Two of the six pleasures came with pregnancy, and suggest that she is finding this phase of parenting has expanded her life in some positive ways. Rachel wants to increase her involvement with the things she values. In her particular case, pregnancy has encouraged doing more of her highest-ranking activities, and has prohibited only one, getting high on alcohol. However, in looking forward to the birth of her baby, she finds that five of six activities will be restricted by having an infant, and three of them will be prohibited for several weeks when the baby is new. She finds that she has not done a good job of valuing herself in fulfilling her desires for swiming, relaxation, and rock climbing, and makes contracts with herself to meet her needs.

She further realizes that dreaming about the baby has value of its own and resolves to stop belittling this activity as useless and a waste of time. She analyzes some of the drawbacks to sobriety and makes plans to reduce them with a little help from her friends. She ranks her most valued activities and discovers she really does not value the old ways of getting high as much as she thought.

She also learns that she needs support from her partner and friends if she is going to actualize pregnancy and survive the early months of parenting with a baby. She decides to open up this topic with Sam and friends with an aim of planning to meet those needs when the time comes.

In general, she finds that pregnancy is not as great a giving to the baby as she thought: she seems to be getting a great deal out of it herself. But she is forewarned that unless she does some work in advance of the baby's arrival, she may find having a new baby "too much giving" and experience unintentional martyrdom.

Companionship Parenthood

In our culture parenthood is in transition from a traditional pattern with rigid roles for parent and child, to a more open, personal relationship based on sharing, communication, and mutual respect. In making this transition, parenthood lags behind the institution of marriage, which is well on the way toward new forms which meet the personal needs of both men and women as individuals. David R. Mace, Ph.D., marriage counselor and cofounder of the

Finally, at age 38 with the third baby, I surprised myself. I could really ask people for things, and they came through. It was a nice experience, and we are closer for it.

My other postpartum times were awful, because I had not planned ahead for specific things, then felt guilty asking, asking, asking. . . .

My mother-in-law came to stay with us when the baby was ten days old. She did a lot of chores for me and I felt guilty. I wanted my husband to do everything so we could be alone, though it was putting an extra burden on him. Contrast that with my attitude a year later: when Grandma arrived, I fell to my knees in gratitude. I had learned that a woman with a small child needs all the help she can get.

Association of Couples for Marriage Enrichment, describes this changing concept of marriage in the *Journal of Marriage and Family Counseling* (April 1976).

> I take the view, shared widely by others, that the traditional marriage, with its rigid institutional character, cannot survive in our new, open society. It is rapidly being replaced by an alternative form, clearly recognized by Ernest Burgess in 1945, and described by him as the companionship marriage . . . [based on] interpersonal relationships, mutual affection, sympathetic understanding, comradeship. The popular terminology would describe it as being based less on duty than on love.

Likewise, in *Pleasure Bond* (Boston: Little, Brown and Co., 1975), William Masters and Virginia Johnson, noted researchers in human sexuality, write of the need to go beyond a commitment to roles as husband and wife into a personal commitment to each other for a true love bond to develop.

We Know the Language of Love All Our Lives

A similar change in the character of parent-child relations receives impetus from demands made by both parents and children. Our culture places a high value on love at all ages. Songs, books, television, movies, advertisements, and so on tell us of the importance of love to personal happiness, so that from the age a child learns to speak, he also learns the language of love. And the language of love he learns is not that of duty but of companionship.

Just as traditional roles of husband and wife thwarted the growth of intimacy and companionship in marriage, traditional roles of parent and child may restrict the development of mutual understanding and a sense of partnership in the family. The deciding factor is whether or not the parent (and later, the child) overcommits him/herself to the parental role and undercommits him/herself as a person.

A father, for example, may accept the role of breadwinner for his children but not know or accept them as individuals. Mothers may find themselves locked into their positions as nurturers and protectors; overmothering and overprotective women are as ignorant of who their children are and as unloving as the father who serves quite adequately as breadwinner, but not as a person. And children, learning by example from their parents, other adults, and their peers, may strengthen and prolong the commit-

I am indeed blessed in the true sense of the word. Our marital relationship is one of constant discovery, growth, and love. I am in excellent health and better shape, figuratively and literally speaking, than I have ever been in my life. And, we have a beautiful, healthy baby.

ment to roles so that the mature family comes to resemble a cast of masked characters more than a group of people.

Traditional roles may serve an important function, however, when they are viewed as a means to achieve companionship parenthood rather than as an end in themselves. Most adults approach parenthood with vague notions of what their parental roles will be. These idealized visions of parental characteristics are apt to be traditional, having been absorbed through contact with one's own parents and other adults. Commitment to an idealized version of motherhood or fatherhood may be an important stage in the development of parents. It is a beginning which eventually matures into the deep fullness of parenting. Most of the joy and satisfaction to be had in parenthood is experienced with a breakthrough from traditional postures into companionship parenthood, with its greater joy and satisfaction.

Er, Hello, Baby

It is even easier to become stuck in the role of "pregnant" than other phases of parenthood. This depersonalizes the relationship with your baby more than in other stages of parenthood. The child seems not to exist and direct communication appears to be impossible.

You can step beyond wondering what your child will be like, however, and begin to know this child of yours. Several authorities have expressed the opinion that babies are individuals in the womb, too, and that, for example, babies who frequently get hiccups from drinking amniotic fluid tend to be rapid eaters with hearty appetites on the outside, as well. Pregnancy has been viewed as a time of passivity and waiting for so long, however, that little work has been done to confirm these observations and describe fetal behavior in relation to mother-and-father behavior and in relation to baby behavior after birth.

It helps, first of all, to get a feel for what the baby's life is like inside. One of the great surprises for us was hearing a recording of sounds in the uterus. We are still trying to recover from the confusion of noise; we cannot believe that babies are not nervous wrecks when they are born. For a beginning acquaintance with your baby read "The Secret World of the Baby," in Day and Liley's 1967 book *Modern Motherhood: Pregnancy, Childbirth, and the Newborn Baby* (New York: Random House, 1967).

Can You Tell What Your Baby Likes?

Try becoming aware of your baby's behavior. Is he/she affected by your moods? Lovemaking? Music? Light or

I kept a dream log throughout my pregnancy. It made me more aware of the strength of my hopes and fears. They were what you'd expect: the baby is beautiful; the baby is strange. I will survive; I may not survive. I found myself fighting back in my dreams when I was worried, and, no doubt, that helped me in reality.

When I was 13, I would put my baby brother to sleep by singing to him as I rocked, but Catherine seems unimpressed by my singing, so we rock in silence most of the time. If I feel good, I sing while we're getting ready for bed; she seems to approve of this.

darkness? Different body positions? Exercise? Times of day or night?

Try communicating with him/her by touch. Is that a hand? Where is the head? What does he/she feel like inside? Massage your baby through the abdominal wall; what does he/she do? When does the baby hiccup? What does he/she do when your uterus contracts? Afterward?

Listen to him/her. Tape-record the sounds of the environment near the womb. Which sounds come from the baby? Which from you? Do these sounds change at various times?

Interact with the baby. Can you make up a game? Will he/she move away from your hand pressing against the abdomen? Will the movements stop, then start again in response to some behavior of yours? Will he/she play versions of Pat-a-Cake from inside? Take him/her for a walk to a favorite place. Introduce him/her to your favorite music.

Talk and sing to the baby. Cradle him/her (and mother) in your arms. Tell stories. Plan trips together, tell what you are thinking and feeling. Share your dreams with your baby.

Record your discoveries about the baby and yourselves, your speculations, dreams, fantasies, the things you do to relate to your baby inside. You can put this record on tape, in journal form, or in letters to be read when the child is older.

A definition of experiment: "A trial made to confirm or disprove something doubtful; an operation undertaken to discover some unknown principle or effect, or to test some suggested truth."

The experimental approach to parenting takes into account the mother's needs to find what is right for herself and her child, recognizing the fact that each one is a unique, changing individual. This method is usual during pregnancy with regard to selecting and asserting one's need for medical care and childbirth education. It's also valuable in reworking relationships with friends and mates, and in developing a lifestyle that meets one's changed needs for sleep and rest, excellent nutrition, exercise, work and play, sexual activity, and so forth.

Selection of medical care is one of the most important areas of pregnant parenting. A poor choice can result in inappropriate medical attention, with effects ranging from unpleasant to disastrous. Yet this is an area where most parents yield their authority and responsibility with appalling ease.

Try applying the experimental approach to your medical care in the column below. As you proceed through steps 1 to 5 in the left-hand column, we will offer comments and suggestions in the right.

By the third baby, I was able to palpate my abdomen to feel the head and the rear and recognize the feet or the hands. I bought a stethoscope to hear the heartbeat. It was exciting to get to know my baby a little more. With my first pregnancy, I don't really believe I thought there was a baby inside.

I kept a chart of the baby's movements for a month. It was entertaining. But on days when I felt no movement I worried, so I stopped keeping the record.

Knowing her now, I'd say her movements in the womb—she was fluid, neither hyperactive nor sluggish—correspond to the way she is in person.

We went to a "big deal" natural childbirth doctor. I waited in his office two to four hours on every prenatal appointment. He spent five minutes with me, patted me on the head every time I asked a question or expressed concern, and told me everything was fine. I felt that since he had such a good reputation, he must know what he was doing and that I was just a bother. I reasoned that it must be boring to answer the same questions that pregnant women ask time and time again—so I was understanding of the doctor's difficulties and I was a "good girl." Just before my birth time arrived, my doctor informed me he was about to retire. He said he would not be coming to the hospital for night births any more, and, of course, we gave birth at night.

Experimental Approach to Seeking Medical Care

1. Become aware of your feelings about your medical care.

A. View prenatal care as an indicator of the care you will receive during labor, birth, and postpartum. Do not accept hasty examinations, unanswered questions, long waits, or lack of interest. Don't put up with the attitude, "Don't you worry about a thing; I'll decide what should be done," with the idea that your care will be better at birth, when it supposedly really counts. First of all, prenatal care has greater influence on a healthy outcome than birth care alone. Just as important, these prenatal visits indicate the medical style of your doctor, midwife, clinic, hospital, or birth center. If you feel you are just another uterus to them now, expect to be the same or less during labor and birth.

2. Question the appropriateness of your present parenting behavior.

B. List your negative and positive feelings after each visit. Look at this list from time to time to see how you stand.

3. Change your behavior.

C. Recall how you selected this particular care giver. Now think of buying something expensive—a car or a house. Did you give equal or more time and effort to selecting your medical support? How many houses did you look at before buying? How many doctors and midwives did you interview, and how many hospitals have you investigated?

4. Note the effects of these changes.

D. Visit the place where you will give birth several times. What is its feel? Draw a picture of it. What is it like? A jail? A factory? A nest?

5. Evaluate and decide to relate to original care provider in new ways, change to a new provider, or accept your negative feelings.

E. With a friend, try this role-play: Instruct your friend to be you, asking questions about birth. You respond as your medical provider usually responds to you. Try this experiment with your friend being in different moods—persistent, shy, angry, forthright, logical.

Afterward, consider how your friends feel about you and your baby being in the hands of this person.

A. Review your responses to step 1, select the negative aspects of your medical care, and resolve to improve them.

A. Try relating to your medical provider in new ways.

1. List your needs and tell him of them.
2. Take your partner or an informed friend who will support you.
3. Let your medical person know what dissatisfies you, and likewise, what you like.
4. If you note resistance, try to understand his feelings, and let him know you are hearing his feelings.
5. Focus on *your* feelings rather than debate obstetrical technique.
6. Offer to research the topic for him (see reading list for help).
7. Arrange your appointments for times when he is more likely to feel free to talk, and let him know that is why you selected those times.

B. Recognize and challenge attitudes that stand in the way of effective questioning: "Doctor knows best," "Pregnancy is out of my hands, but wait until the baby is born," "All doctors and hospitals are alike," "I'm so turned on—or tired out—by pregnancy, I just don't have the interest (time, strength) to really do a good job of selecting medical care," "I'm not competent to decide what is good care and what is not," "Pregnancy, that's woman's work."

B. List your needs and arrange consultations with other medical people until you find one who suits you. For leads, contact hospitals and ask the obstetrical nurse for names of some doctors who support natural or prepared childbirth, La Leche League, the International Childbirth Education Association, and local childbirth and breastfeeding groups. Consultations are less expensive than regular medical appointments. They are for discussion only and do not involve a medical examination.

C. Read to increase your awareness of the wide range of parenting choices regarding medical care.

C. Investigate unconventional medical services such as out-of-hospital birth centers, home birth, hospital, and midwifery services.

D. Join a consumer-oriented childbirth education class or other group heavily committed to expanding the options open to parents during pregnancy and birth.

I had to hide the fact that we were planning a home birth from the doctor in order to obtain prenatal care. The local physicians have pressured any colleagues sympathetic to the idea of home birth into refusing prenatal care; all this accomplishes is to contribute to potential complications at home. I don't think it deters anyone who wants a home birth to have a doctor refuse them prenatal care. They go to a public clinic or just "forget" to mention their plans.

I had to have three stitches after birth and we went to the hospital to have it done. My doctor (who was a woman, incidentally) was furious when she found out we had given birth at home, and she called in a nurse from the hospital to witness her bawling us out! She wanted a backup person to prove that she had not knowingly cooperated with us by seeing me during my pregnancy. Now she wants us to pay her almost her complete fee even though she did not attend the birth!

In our area the pressure against home birth is so strong that the hospital will revoke a doctor's admitting privileges if she/he willingly participates in a nonemergency birth outside the hospital.

I never planned to have another pregnancy but this marriage changed all that. This time it was so exciting because we had a united interest in our developing baby.

Review step 1, suggestions a. through e. Compare your responses to these same activities now with your earlier responses. What has made you feel better about the quality of your medical care? Worse? More realistic? Accepting?

a. Do not hesitate to change health care providers because you have already paid a large amount of money to the original one; he should charge you for your visits but refund the rest. Also, do not hesitate because of nearness of due date, unless the provider you are switching to refuses to take you for this reason; closeness to due date is not a risk factor.

b. Most pregnant parents find it very difficult to switch medical persons due to feelings of loyalty, fears of being embarrassed or insulted, making the doctor angry, the possibility of some form of reprisal from the doctor or hospital at a later date, or feelings of guilt at being disobedient and a rebel. It helps to be aware through reading or conversation with other parents of the intense anger, guilt, humiliation, sorrow, and actual physical damage that may result when parents act counter to their feelings about medical persons.

The Pleasure Concept

"The giving and the receiving of pleasure is a need and an ecstasy."—Kahlil Gibran, *The Prophet* (New York: Alfred Knopf, 1923).

Parenting encompasses many pleasures—sex, play, breastfeeding, sharing, accomplishment, personal growth, touching, cuddling, talking and singing, visual beauty, smells, and loving—and these pleasures bond man, woman, and child so that a wide range of needs, including those related to survival, personal growth, and finding meaning in life, can be met. Pleasure is essential to effective parenting.

Unfortunately, the Puritan ethic lingers, and pleasure tends to be overlooked as a wholly legitimate and necessary concern of parents. Conventional social forms during the perinatal period, for example, restrict the couple's access to sex (commonly prohibited for extended periods); to sharing pregnancy, birth, and early parenting (men generally are discouraged from participation, and many women are limited to the passive role of patient); play (the attitude that pregnancy is a fragile condition); touching and cuddling (these activities are often linked to sexual activity so that couples engage in them less as they decrease purely sexual interaction); talking ("What's to talk about, with her wrapped up in the baby?" "What's to talk about, he wouldn't understand."); and breastfeeding (still misunderstood and neglected by the bulk of the medical establishment). Under the prevailing cultural atmosphere, it is no wonder that the arrival of a child is usually something in the nature of a disaster for the marriage that conceived it.

According to J. Richard Udry, author of *The Social Context of Marriage*, 3rd ed. (Philadelphia: J.B. Lippincott Co., 1974), research indicates that children generally hasten the disengagement of husband and wife from their marriage relationship. However, we doubt that this withdrawal from marriage with the coming of children is inevitable; instead, we think that our cultural pattern for launching families is primarily responsible for the destructive effects the arrival of children has on marriage. In a 1977 article for *Keeping Abreast Journal*, we wrote about what happens to marriage in typical perinatal experience.

Before (the first) pregnancy, a man and woman usually share a companionate relationship and a love marked by play, a sense of happiness, self-confidence, self-reliance, and an active involvement in their joint life. Their relationship overshadows others, such as relationships at work. Based on their successful experience with each other, the couple decides to create a family, or to accept pregnancy. If it can be said that the (prepregnancy) period sets the stage for the perinatal period, and that together these early stages of married life affect the outcome of marriage and parenthood in the long run, then the outlook for the typical couple is rosy. One would expect their marriage to be satisfying and parenthood to be a joint endeavor carried out with enthusiasm and with high rewards to both parents.

But something goes wrong in the perinatal stage. They emerge from the experience a different couple than they were when they decided to become parents. Their attitudes in relation to others change; now they are receptive to the advice of others outside their marriage, passive, unsure of themselves, apt to form strong attachments to others outside marriage, such as the pregnant woman's attachment to her doctor. They are disengaged from the marital relationship, less companionate in their approach to marriage, and far more absorbed in conventional roles as breadwinner and mother than in each other.

Marriage no longer means play. The pleasure bond was weakened during the experiences of pregnancy, birth, and early parenting, all of which are associated in the couple's minds with duty, sickness, even tempo-

I was knowledgeable of the Lamaze method from friends who were enthusiastic about their experience. Jim was open to this, so we found a Lamaze teacher and attended the six-week preparation. Jim encouraged me to do my exercises, and we practiced the breathing, working especially hard during the last month. The teaching connected with Lamaze, for example, of the physical aspects of pregnancy, the development of the baby, the effects of drugs, plus the practice and togetherness of the method itself were invaluable to us and to the birth of Rachael.

Besides Lamaze, we attended a four-week Red Cross class for parents-to-be. We were the oldest couple there! This class was a great help in providing practical suggestions and reading matter which helped me to care for my baby after birth.

We also toured the maternity facilities of the hospital where Rachael was to be born. Besides becoming familiar with the surroundings, we wanted to let the personnel know that we were a Lamaze couple.

rary insanity. Marriage is no longer rewarding in itself; rewards have been postponed indefinitely.

In summary, our cultural pattern for the perinatal experience appears to demolish what foundations the couple has established in the events leading up to conception: the sharing, commitment, the sense of being special, the mutual pleasuring, the high degree of self-reliance as a couple.

Make It a Rewarding Joint Endeavor

My husband caught his son, showing a super high elation I had never before seen in a man. His pride was indescribable. He cut and clamped the cord and weighed the baby after the first nursing. I wish I had tape-recorded the birth to pick up my husband's elation at the time of birth. The relationship between father and son has stayed very close.

Having participated actively in the plans for and actual labor of the birth of our son we really enjoyed a relaxed first birth.

Our beautiful birth was also shared by my husband's mother who had experienced only drugged deliveries. She said our son's birth was the most beautiful thing she'd ever witnessed.

Investigations of exceptions to the general rule bear out these observations and indicate that active, educated, shared mother-father participation in perinatal events is pleasurable and does serve as a basis for perceiving parenthood as a personally rewarding joint endeavor. In her book, *Why Natural Childbirth?* (New York: Doubleday, 1972), Dr. Deborah Tanzer wrote about joint participation in childbirth within a hospital setting. She found that wives with husbands present and actively supporting them in labor and birth more often found birth to be an uplifting peak experience, saw themselves in more positive ways, and perceived their husbands as competent, caring men. Several other investigators have shown that husbands who share the experience of birth with their wives gain in self-esteem, see their wives more positively, and feel closer to their infants.

These parents stand in stark contrast to the majority, whose passive, uneducated, rather lonely approach to childbearing is reflected in common attitudes that parenting is unrewarding, a burden to be endured, and ultimately resented and fled from.

By responding differently to pregnancy, birth, and postpartum, parents may avoid weakening their relationship and strengthen it instead. One of the key factors is the giving and receiving of pleasure that goes on throughout the perinatal period.

Sexual Activity

One of the primary sources of mutual pleasuring for most couples is sex, with the focus on sexual intercourse. Many pleasures are engaged in during sexual activity—play, sharing, touching, holding, talking, appreciation of sight and smell—in addition to purely sexual activities. Sex encompasses a large number of needs, is a powerful bonding force and a joy, all at the same time.

But sexual activity often declines significantly during pregnancy and the first months after birth, and parents lose the pleasures, the bonding, and the solace they have learned to find in sex. Although couples have been, and continue to be, urged to expect this decline, even to consider it normal and, therefore, one of the prices pregnant and new parents must pay, a decrease in sexual activity adds stress to the marital and to the parental relationship.

In a 1966 report to the American Psychiatric Association, Meyerowitz and Feldman noted that "the area of sexual adjustment was the leading specific cause of complaint between the spouses," during the transition to parenthood. The withdrawal from sex has even more detrimental impact when it is the primary bonding force between man and woman, as it may be for many couples. In these relationships, disengagement from sexual activity may pull the foundation out from under the relationship.

An unfortunate mixture of medical and cultural misinformation exerts a powerful second force on couples to decrease or abstain from sexual activity, in most cases, unnecessarily. Nurse-midwife Lonnie Holtzman reported in "Sexual Practices During Pregnancy," *Journal of Nurse-Midwifery* (Spring, 1976):

Medical research and literature do not substantiate the common practice of arbitrarily curtailing sexual activity in the normal female. Physicians and nurse-midwives often impose sexual limitations on their patients ranging from early pregnancy to the last trimester of pregnancy.

In my study, it was clear that many patients were given false information, limited information, or no information about sexual activity during pregnancy. Only 60 percent of the patients had any recommendations about sexual intercourse made to them. Even when recommendations were made, the quality of these recommendations was limited. One patient was told, "If you feel the need, you can engage in sexual intercourse; but it would be best not to." Another patient, who was having a normal antepartum course, was told not to have any sex during pregnancy because she had had a previous miscarriage. This patient reported spontaneous orgasms in her sleep and suffered from severe guilt feelings about these orgasms. She stated to me, "I really couldn't stop them; it just happened—it was in my sleep. Thank God they didn't hurt my baby." Other patients had sexual limitations placed on them as early as the 28th week of pregnancy, although these patients were having normal antepartum courses.

With my first pregnancy, my husband and I were told, "No sexual activity from about six weeks before the due date until about six weeks after." And we obeyed that edict! How trusting we were, and how we suffered through those weeks of abstinence.

Not this time—never before had I felt so sexually alive. My body responded to this pregnancy with intensely heightened physical pleasures. Our sexual activities increased. Lovemaking became a constantly sought joy and it also enabled us to further share our wonder and pleasure at my ever-changing body. It was truly a celebration of life and love.

Contraindications to sexual intercourse during pregnancy do exist. There is no doubt that threatened abortion in the first trimester, impending miscarriage, premature rupture of the membrances, bleeding, or pain in the later months of pregnancy are indications that medical attention is necessary, and that coital precautions should be exercised.

The patients in my study unanimously reported questions on whether sexual intercourse was really permissible during pregnancy. Both males and females curtailed sexual activity during pregnancy, because they feared injury to the conceptus. This type of misinformation should be dispelled by the physician and the nurse-midwife. Patients are entitled to the real facts concerning the effects of sexual contact during pregnancy.

Where there is legitimate medical concern about miscarriage, couples need to be aware that maternal orgasm produces uterine contractions, so that the mother will refrain from masturbation as well as intercourse. There is also one particular sexual practice, that of blowing air into the vagina, that is dangerous, especially during the latter part of pregnancy and before the uterus is completely healed after birth. In a few cases, this practice is believed to have caused air embolism (an air bubble circulating through the blood), which can be fatal.

Clearly, these legitimate restrictions on sexual activity are a far cry from the blanket prohibitions on sex starting anytime from early pregnancy to the seventh or eighth month and continuing until the sixth week postpartum or later that have prevailed for the past several decades, and should constitute little interference with the lovemaking of most couples. In the absence of medical contraindications, most forms of sexual activity are considered both safe and desirable throughout pregnancy until labor begins and may be resumed at three to four weeks after birth, information for which pregnant couples may breath a grateful sigh of relief.

Our bedrock cultural belief seems to be that sex during pregnancy and after is, or may be, dangerous. In the absence of adequate knowledge to the contrary, couples tend to feel fearful, confused, frustrated, and guilty, and gradually decrease their sexual contact. The impossibility of enjoying sex while engaged in emotional turmoil of this nature may go a long way toward explaining the gradual decline in sexual activity that is typical of most couples.

The final and ultimately crucial element in perinatal sexual decline is the partners themselves. Their feelings, thoughts, communication, concern, and effort determine the outcome of sexual pleasuring.

Discoveries

Most of these reasons for avoiding sex will diminish provided couples get accurate information, openly share their feelings and thoughts, and make a joint effort to enrich their sexual relationship. But this is easier said than done. Masters and Johnson write of women who refrained

Pregnancy	Postpartum
fear of injuring the baby	crying baby
recommendations by physician	sleepless nights, exhaustion
loss of interest	spouting nipples
physical discomfort	sore perineum (area between the vagina and rectum)
awkwardness	
loss of attractiveness	fear of harm to woman
mate's apprehension	overwhelming physical and emotional involvement of woman in care of baby
fear of injuring the woman	
introspection of woman	
kicking fetus	depression
dripping breasts	sore breasts
fatigue	tight vagina (too many stitches taken after episiotomy)
nausea (early pregnancy)	
maternal fear of her own increased sexual drive (three to six months pregnant)	doctor's orders (prohibition on sex for six weeks after birth)
	tension
mixed feelings about the woman's growing motherliness	flabby stomach
	lochia (discharge)
	fear of waking baby
	feelings of emotional distance as result of the above

from sex after childbirth because they feared physical damage, but who did not discuss this with their partners nor seek better understanding of the physiological facts. Other women reported experiencing sexual arousal while breastfeeding which led them to feel guilty. They did not realize that breastfeeding, intercourse, and childbirth are closely interconnected forms of female sexual behavior, and it is natural that where one is experienced as sexually pleasurable, the others may well be, too.

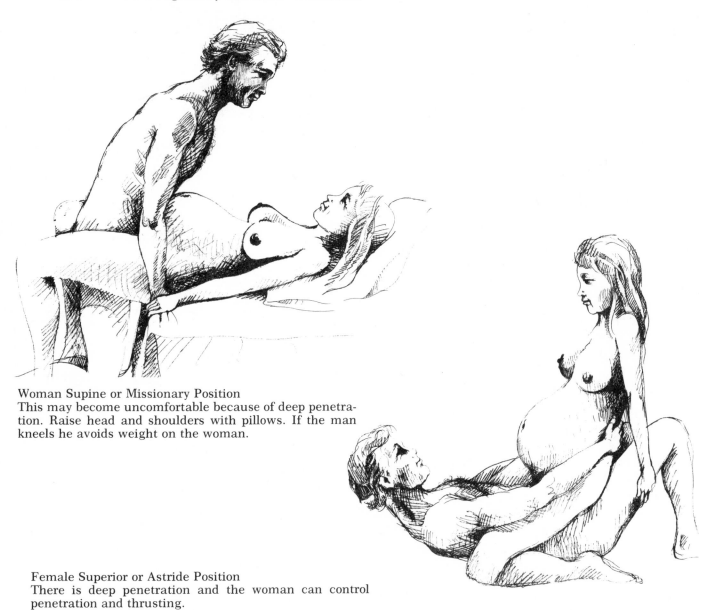

Woman Supine or Missionary Position
This may become uncomfortable because of deep penetration. Raise head and shoulders with pillows. If the man kneels he avoids weight on the woman.

Female Superior or Astride Position
There is deep penetration and the woman can control penetration and thrusting.

Side or Lateral Position (as seen from above)
There is less penetration and the woman has more freedom of movement.

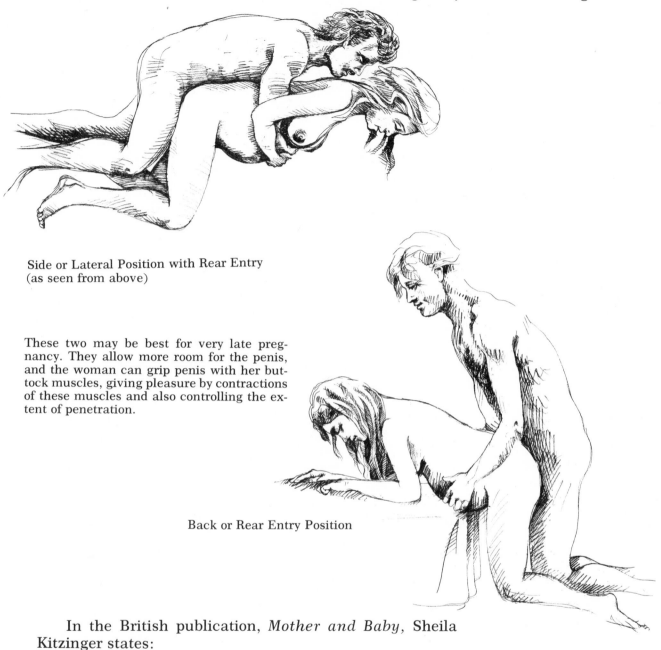

Side or Lateral Position with Rear Entry
(as seen from above)

These two may be best for very late pregnancy. They allow more room for the penis,
and the woman can grip penis with her but-
tock muscles, giving pleasure by contractions
of these muscles and also controlling the extent of penetration.

Back or Rear Entry Position

In the British publication, *Mother and Baby*, Sheila
Kitzinger states:

Pregnancy is an ideal time for husband and wife to
embark on a journey of discovery into the mystery of
each other's bodies and the patterns of response in
which each take delight. The unborn child, far from
being an intruder in the marriage, brings with it the
opportunity for a new tenderness.

Some discoveries will involve changes in coital position.
Breasts may feel full, tender, and especially responsive to
fingertip and oral caresses during pregnancy. However, this
sensitivity can result in pain with too much pressure,

overstimulation, and roughness. Sheila Kitzinger points out the need for flexibility in sexual response, too.

> If pregnancy is advanced, it may also be better for the husband to ejaculate just before the woman enters the phase of accelerated rhythmic movements that result in orgasm. This may seem odd advice when books stress that the man must wait, but she may be unable to embark on free movement of her pelvis and the pelvic floor musculature when the penis is still erect and rigid inside her. Thus hampered in her movements, the chances of her reaching orgasm are reduced. So it may be best for the husband to ejaculate first, and then, with caresses (or otherwise), to lead his wife onwards to her own orgasm.

Clearly, flexibility of this sort depends on open discussion of each individual's needs and feelings.

Following birth, many couples do not wait the prescribed four to six weeks to resume sexual relations. It is important that the uterus be healed, however, to avoid the possibility of uterine infection. Masters and Johnson, in *Human Sexuality,* report that women are usually physically fit for intercourse about a week after the baby is born. Couples who desire to resume intercourse earlier than the traditional time can speed matters up by breastfeeding, which hastens involution of the uterus (return to nonpregnant size and shape) and by arranging for an earlier postpartum check to verify healing. There are reports that some obstetricians encourage renewed sexual activity as early as three weeks after birth if the couple desires and physical factors are normal.

Maternal Exhaustion as an Obstacle to Lovemaking

Couples may find that maternal exhaustion, one of the primary obstacles to lovemaking at this time, can be reduced by planning each day on paper to take advantage of baby's nap-times as times for mother to sleep; to create realistic goals for housekeeping, cooking, and other necessities (rule of thumb: the lower the goal, the more realistic the goal); to get help when and where it is available; and to find the time of least fatigue and tension for lovemaking. Soreness, another big handicap to passion, can be minimized by avoiding an unnecessary episiotomy (cut in the perineum, purportedly made to ease the process of birth), relaxation of the pelvic floor (Kegel or pubococcygeal) muscles at penetration, use of extra lubrication to counter the vaginal dryness which often follows birth, and coital positions which put the pressure of the penis on the front part of the vagina rather than the tender area at the back where the cut for the episiotomy was made (if it was).

Kitzinger adds: "It is often much better for the wife to help the husband inside, so that she does not feel the need to recoil like a snail drawing in its horns. As he slides in, she should deliberately release all her pelvic floor muscles so that they are suspended downwards like a heavy hammock."

Breast-feeding mothers may find their breasts especially sensitive at night when the baby may be sleeping longer. Gentleness and variations in position may be called for to avoid discomfort here as well.

There is a set of muscles, variously called the pelvic floor, Kegel, or pubococcygeal muscles, that are often undeveloped in women but which play a large part in sexual functioning and physical and emotional health. These muscles surround the urethra, the vagina, and the anus in a three-ringed eight shape. When they contract they close all three openings, and when they relax they open all three. Good muscle tone is important in preventing uterine prolapse (sagging of the uterus and bladder), and stress incontinence (involuntary urination and defecation).

Learning to relax and tighten these muscles at will enables a woman to ease the process of birth and lessens the likelihood of perineal tearing. It also acts to lessen the soreness sometimes involved in resuming sex after birth as Sheila Kitzinger describes above. It works to add to the pleasure of sex throughout pregnancy and for the rest of her days by using these muscles to grip and caress the penis.

A New Focus on Sexual Pleasuring

Personal reasons for decreasing sex during the perinatal period may persist in spite of the best information, communication, planning, cooperation, and technique. This does not mean that the couple must forgo the benefits of mutual pleasuring. Traditional solutions to this dilemma which separates man and woman—cold showers, avoiding each other, hard liquor, tranquilizers, the father finding someone else for the duration—are not the answer. A new perspective on sexual pleasuring is required which replaces the focus on intercourse and orgasm with an emphasis on mutual pleasuring: touching, holding, talking, sharing, and play. These pleasures are enjoyed by couples during sexual activity and are needlessly lost when sex declines during the perinatal period. These other forms of pleasuring are less intense than sexual orgasm, but they are extremely

Our old-fashioned herbal, food, and vitamin home remedies really worked wonders on my sore and tender vaginal area. About 2½ weeks after our baby was born, we decided to very gingerly try lovemaking. With much delicacy and gentleness, our love transpired. Much to our surprise and chagrin, we discovered that we had unnecessarily waited too long! I felt good inside and responded as ever. I suppose this could be regarded as an added benefit to a truly natural home birth with proper prenatal and postpartum care.

powerful in their own right and can as effectively meet the same needs for tension release, expansion of intimacy and mutuality, and physical pleasure as the most passionate sexual encounter, without the imposition of demands for sexual intercourse.

In *What Now? A Handbook for New Parents* (New York: Charles Scribner's Sons, 1975), a book about surviving the postpartum period, Barbara Banet and Mary Lou Rozdilsky write:

I'm thinking about when you feel like making love and I don't—usually that is a Bad Scene. I am closed, tight, and that makes me feel awful. How could I possibly give anything when I feel like that? Then one day I got a glimpse of something new: I didn't feel like making love but I was really caring about you, wanting to make you feel good. I lit some candles and put on a record we both like. I said, "Roll over," and I gave you a fantastic back rub—pounding, caressing, letting my long hair trail over your bare back. I put my cheek on your back, my nose, my ear, my lips. I rubbed the tight muscles at the base of your neck. I traced a pattern there. It makes sense that you would rather have a back rub freely and joyfully given than make love to a body without a soul in it. I must admit, a cup of hot tea (with honey and lemon, even) won't always satisfy a man who wants to make love. But a funny thing happens, sometimes, when I am free to give what I want to give at the moment; it opens me up, makes me feel like a human being again—and who knows what might happen then?"

As she says, "Who knows what might happen then?" For couples whose sexual activity is in a decline, not for physical or medical reasons, pleasuring may do more than substitute for sex; it may revive their interest in it. Sexual response cannot be forced. Reasons for not being interested in sex other than physical and medical ones are valid. Sex freely given is a joy; sex given under pressure is both a burden and a source of disaffection that may well destroy a relationship. As Masters and Johnson point out, arousal in both man and woman occurs when the individual receives sexual stimuli, but that reception of these stimuli can be blocked by becoming distracted during sexual activity. The therapeutic approach described in *Human Sexual Inadequacy* (Boston: Little, Brown and Co., 1970) seeks to circumvent distraction and its inevitable blocking effect by encouraging couples to focus not on sexual performance but rather on pleasuring. Only after pleasuring leads to arousal are couples slowly led from pleasuring to full sexual activity.

To a degree, couples experiencing a decline in sexual interest during the perinatal period share this pattern. Perhaps most of the reasons listed in Table 1 could constitute sufficient distraction to inhibit arousal. These distractions block the couple's psychophysiological response to sexual stimuli and they lose interest. Sex becomes a matter of performance or work instead of play. By changing the emphasis from sexual intercourse to one of giving and receiving pleasure, couples may find some of their old interest in sex returning. However, this approach requires that couples truly focus on pleasuring and not have a hidden agenda aimed at using the pleasuring activity to guarantee sexual arousal. One activity most people find very enjoyable is massage.

Massage: a Loving Touch

You don't need any familiarity with formal anatomy to give a good body massage. Nor do you need the Herculean hands of a burly Swedish masseur. And all that's needed in the way of equipment is some padding to lay on the floor and some vegetable oil.

The first instruction is: Don't use your bed for massage. A bed is too soft to provide a firm enough support. So instead of bouncing around on a Beautyrest, take two or three blankets, fold them lengthwise on the floor, and cover them with a sheet. You can also use foam as a padding or move a single mattress onto the floor. But whatever padding you use, make sure it's at least an inch or two thick, and it should be wide and long enough so that when your partner lies down, there's still room for you to sit or kneel to one side.

Also, you might want to turn off the overhead light; both the atmosphere and your partner will be more relaxed. Bright light that falls directly on the face causes eye muscles to tense.

Keep the room warm and free of drafts. George Downing, author of *The Massage Book* (New York: Random House, 1972), cautions that "nothing destroys an otherwise good massage more quickly than physical coldness." If your spouse begins to feel cold, use a spare sheet to cover the body parts that you're not working on at the moment.

Now prepare the oil. Why use oil at all? Without a lubricating agent, your hands can't really apply enough pressure and still move smoothly over the skin. When applying oil, put about a half-teaspoon into your palm, and then spread it smoothly on your partner's skin. Keep the oil near you during the massage; a shallow bowl makes a handy container. Cover the entire surface area you're about to massage—arm, leg, hand, or back—with a barely visible film. Don't use peanut or corn oil. Sesame and olive oil are the easiest to wash out of sheets and clothes. Mix in a few drops of essences such as clove, cinnamon, lemon, rosemary, or camomile to scent the oil.

A Few General Hints

Before you actually use specific strokes, here are a few general hints. Keep your hands relaxed. Also, apply pressure. You'll probably discover that your partner wants quite a bit more pressure than you had expected. But use the weight of your whole body to apply pressure rather than just the muscles of your hands.

Experiment with all the different ways of moving your hands that you can think of. Move them in long strokes. Move them in circles. Explore the structure of the bone and muscle. Move slowly, then speed up your tempo. Or use only your fingertips, pressing them firmly against the muscles or brushing them lightly over the skin. Gently slap, or tap. Ask your partner for feedback: Is that enough pressure? Does that feel good?

While you're taking care of your partner, don't forget to take care of yourself. Keep your back straight whenever possible. And don't worry about how much or how little you do. You'll be moving and positioning your body in many new ways; if you don't take care of yourself, you'll end up with sore muscles. For now, concentrate on one or two body parts at a time.

The massage is arranged in a particular order, but you should start wherever you want. If you decide to work on more than a single part, apply more oil each time you move to a new area.

Finally, try to minimize the amount of turning over that your partner has to do. (It's easiest to work on the arms, hands, feet, and neck while your partner is lying face up.)

Let's start with the back, for the back is the most important part of a massage. The spine is the stalk of the central nervous system, and often anxiety and nervous tension are caused by nothing more than tight, sore muscles around the spine.

First, straddle your partner's thighs. It's the easiest way to work on the back.

Now put your hands on the lower back with the fingertips pointing toward the spine. Move your hands straight up the back. When you get to the top of the back, separate your hands and bring them over the shoulder blades to the floor, and then pull them back down along the sides. Do this stroke four to six times.

Now work with your thumbs on the lower back. Use the balls of your thumbs, and make short, rapid strokes away from you toward the head. Work close to the spine just below the waistline, first on the left side and then on the right. Now put both hands on one hip with your fingers pointing straight down. Pull each hand alternately straight up from the floor, working up to the armpit and then back again. With each stroke, begin pulling one hand just before the other is about to finish so that there is no break between strokes. Do both sides.

Now move to the upper back. Knead the muscles that curve from your partner's neck onto his or her shoulders. Work these muscles gently between the thumb and fingers.

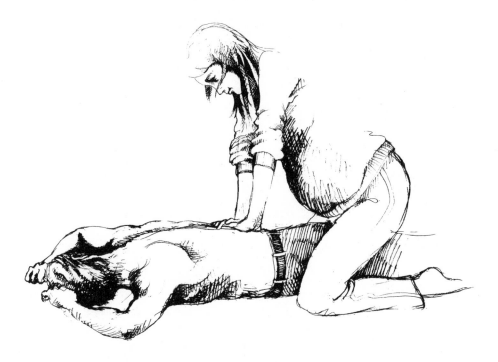

Now use your thumbs on the upper back just as you did on the lower back.

Finally, take the heel of your hand and place it at the base of the spine. Gently press and release, moving little by little up the spine to the neck.

The Effleurage Stroke

Now that you've finished the back, ask your partner to turn over so that you can massage the arms. But first, we'll learn a new stroke: the effleurage.

Place your hands together, one hand on top of the other and thumbs interlinked. When you move your hands, make your strokes long, flowing and unbroken, and put your weight on the heels of your hands rather than on the fingertips. This is an effleurage.

First, effleurage the entire arm from the wrist to the shoulder, taking your hands up over the shoulder and down the side of the arm.

Now massage the inside of the wrist with the balls of your thumbs. Work your hands downward until you have covered all the muscles lying along the inside of the forearm.

Now place your partner's hand on his or her chest. Work from the elbow to the shoulder with the balls of your thumbs, paying particular attention to the muscles on the top of the arm.

Return your partner's arm to his or her side.

Now explore and massage the shoulder joint with your fingers. And end with another effleurage of the entire arm.

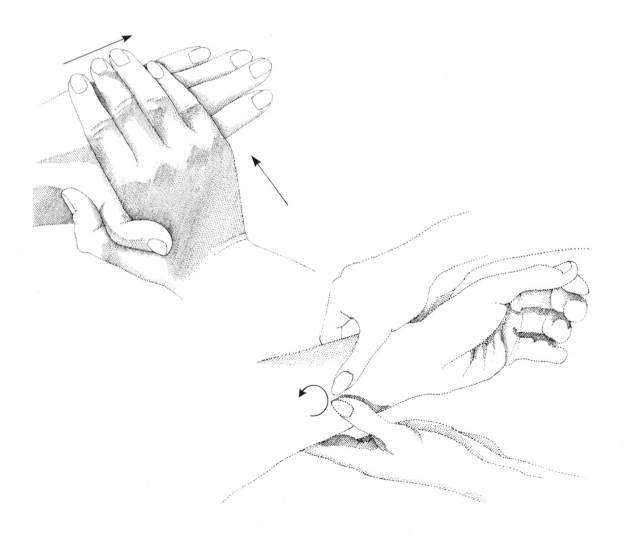

Soothing Strokes for the Browbeaten

Now let's go on to the head. Don't apply any oil to the face before you begin; just put a few drops on your fingertips. Massage the forehead just below the hairline with the balls of your thumbs. Start from the center of the forehead and glide both thumbs at once in either direction. Continue to the temples; now move your thumbs in a small circle. Repeat this stroke until you have covered the whole forehead—your last stroke should run just above your partner's eyebrows.

Cover the forehead with the entire left hand, heel toward one temple, fingertips toward the other. Press down. Now using the right hand, slowly and evenly add more pressure until maximum pressure is reached (your partner will tell you if it's too much). Hold for ten seconds, then release very slowly. Massage lore has it that this stroke can be used to cure a nagging headache.

Now that you've smoothed your partner's harried brow, move on to another area of tension on the face: the jaw. Lightly grasp the tip of the chin between the tips of the

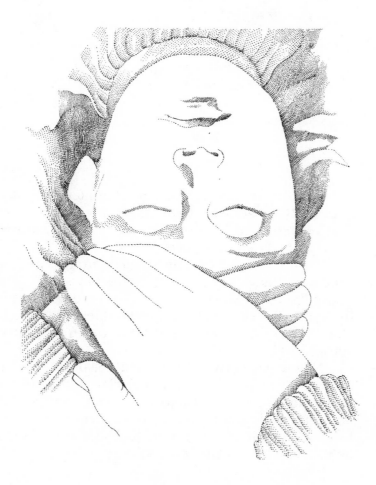

thumb and forefinger of each hand. Follow the edges of the jaw until you have almost reached the ears, and then glide the forefingers into a small circle on the temples. Do this stroke three times.

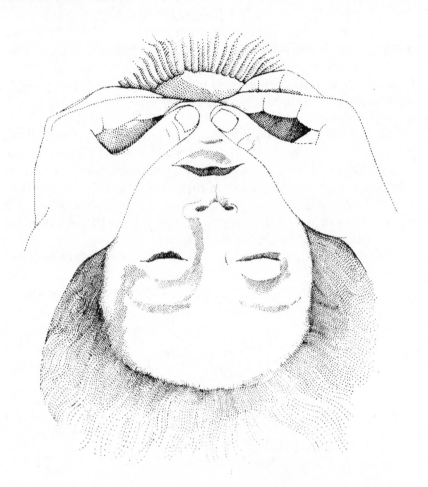

Most of us have neck and shoulder muscles that are habitually tense—so much so, that we don't even realize they're tight and bunched up. That's why loosening these muscles feels so very good.

First massage in egg-shaped circles just above the shoulder blades. Face your palms upward as you work under the body. Start at the outer shoulders, work in toward the spine, then back along the shoulders. You might want to change the direction, speed, and width of your circles as you go.

Now work between the shoulder blades and the spine. Move your fingertips in small circles. Then put your hands under the back of your partner's head, gently lift it a little, and turn it slightly to the left until it rests easily in your left hand. Massage the neck with your free hand. Then turn the head and work on the other side.

Just by working with these simple instructions, you'll soon begin to realize massage's many benefits. Not only does it make you feel good, but it also improves circulation and can relax muscle spasms. Massage often proves useful in relieving fatigue and tension, and is a wonderful way to express affection.

One caution: Do *not* do a lot of massage right away. Rather, do a little at a time and gradually, if you care to, work up to a whole body massage. Begin by working on those parts which are especially sore and stiff.

Massaging your children is a fine idea. Most parents touch only their child's hand or head or feet, but children, too, love to be touched all over.

Whether you make massage a daily event or reserve it for those special romantic evenings, rest assured a tender touch is a gift that is both a joy to give and to receive.

Postpartum Crisis

Each phase of parenting, as of human life as a whole, holds the seeds of the next phase. In addition to its present, each phase has a past and a future. The prechild stage of marriage provides a psychosocial structure which leads to conception and pregnancy. Pregnancy establishes a pattern of parenting and coping as a family that influences the postpartum behavior of the unit, and so on through each stage of the family life cycle. Several writers have observed that parents who postpone having children seem to have more difficulty than others in making the transition from pregnant parenting to parenting the baby. Whether this is a real difference does not much matter because most parents, deferring or not, find the first six weeks or so of living with a baby a time of crisis.

The postpartum crisis, as it is called, has many causes. Recovery from giving birth is one cause and may include persistent fatigue, physical and hormonal changes, soreness and stiffness, emotional sensitivity, and depression. A tremendous sense of responsibility crashes down on most parents as they fully awaken to the fact that a tiny, helpless human being depends entirely on them for life and love. This realization usually leads to feelings of inadequacy which in turn create a frantic urge to learn everything necessary to meet their infant's every need.

Coping with a baby's cries and other noises is a new and nerve-wracking experience in its own right. Babies' cries were designed to evoke a strong response in parents, and they do. But learning what those cries and other noises mean, what to do about them, and when one is adding to the infant's distress rather than helping him takes time and effort during a period when these are in short supply. Added to this is the strain on father and mother in their relationship as a couple.

The postpartum crisis comes unexpectedly to most new parents because they have no prior exposure. This struggle to cope with physical recovery from birth, the new baby, and our adult selves is hidden from public view behind four walls. The many strong emotions this experience elicits—anger, frustration, depression, confusion, fear, guilt—are not those parents are inclined to acknowledge and discuss with others, since to do so would run counter to socially approved behavior for parents and constitute an admission of failure. Also, most parents are so absorbed in surviving that they do not share the experience with others and, in fact, do not have much contact with others outside the home during this time.

Lack of exposure to parenting of new babies leads to naiveté and deficient preparation during pregnancy, which compound the stressfulness of postpartum parenting considerably. This naiveté and its consequences are shown in these statements of two mothers, both in their mid-30s.

Well, I know Hal is looking forward to being a father and I am excited about the baby, too. I don't see the baby making much difference to our marriage, except that we'll have more to share. And if there is a conflict once in a while, the baby can wait a few minutes. I've read that there won't be as much time for housekeeping; I'll have to be less compulsive about cleaning everything, but I think I'll be able to ignore a lot. I'm really looking forward to doing more around the apartment, too.
—Head maternity nurse in a metropolitan hospital, seven months pregnant.

I felt very hemmed in. I was used to being very active and tried to be as active after the birth as before and found that impossible. I felt a very definite pull between my work and spending time with the baby—so consequently tried to schedule my work during times when the baby was sleeping and tried to be up with the baby when he was awake. Of course that was impossible, and I ran myself ragged and experienced all the postnatal problems related to fatigue and always running behind.

Then there was the problem with my husband's and my relationship. Our relationship previously had been built on doing things together—jogging, swimming, theatre, dance, going to concerts and movies. We were never at home together. I couldn't keep up with

I tried to continue going to school with my infant. He was taken care of during class time only, and I did homework while he was asleep. It was too much. My husband was being neglected, and I couldn't give my schoolwork my usual energy. I have taken a leave of absence to get myself together and to enjoy my child. It is so difficult learning to live with a messy house, being tired most of the time, not being able to do anything without interruption, and just being homebound most of the time. Even so, I don't like leaving my child with babysitters, but I'm going to have to discipline myself to do it.

that either and it felt awful—I was very lonely and disturbed about our relationship.

My husband, I think, felt that now I was a mother and he wanted certain things from me—like dinner—I just couldn't cope with that, either.

Our apartment was very small and difficult to manage and not safe for a toddler. Moving was a very financially scary thing for us to do—that was difficult, too.

—Speech therapist, mother of three.

Parents having their first child when they're over 30 may be more isolated with their negative feelings than younger parents, because they are less apt to have friends who have infants, and they may have lost one or more of their own parents.

Plan Ahead for the Postpartum Crisis

The before-after double take is fairly typical. Apparently, pregnancy and birth seize the pregnant parent's attention and do not let go long enough for her to see parenting as the continuum that it is. One mother commented that this obsession with birth and blindness to parenting the newborn is like paying more attention to the gate than to what lies beyond.

There is hope, however. Several writers have described ways parents have softened the transition from pregnant parenting to baby parenting, including: reading, attending classes, arranging for help, joining groups made up of new parents, limiting other commitments during the critical first six weeks, setting aside special times for intimate talk and pleasuring, scheduling time for each parent to be alone, freezing meals ahead of time, sharing parenting tasks whenever possible, deciding on priorities ahead of time, and so on.

Gordon, Kapostin, and Gordon developed a set of guidelines for pregnant parents to use in planning ahead for the postpartum crisis. They appeared in *Journal of Obstetrics and Gynecology* (25: 185, 1965).

- Get help from husband and dependable friends and relatives.
- Make friends of other couples who are experienced with child rearing.
- Don't overload yourself with unimportant tasks.
- Don't move soon after the baby arrives.
- Don't be overconcerned with keeping up appearances.
- Get plenty of rest and sleep.
- Don't be a nurse to relatives or others at this period.
- Confer and consult with husband, family, and experienced friends, and discuss your plans and worries.
- Don't give up outside interests, but cut down on responsibilities and rearrange schedules.

Parenting begins with pregnancy, whether parents recognize the fact or not. The quality of parenting done during pregnancy affects both physical and psychological outcomes of pregnancy. It is probably more important to the well-being of parent, child, and family than any other single factor. However, the importance of parenting during pregnancy is often overlooked or misunderstood and cast in a minor, supporting role. For pregnant parenting to fulfill its potential for creating healthy, happy families, parents must assume responsibility for actualizing pregnancy in all its facets for themselves.

Postpartum Crisis Survival Plan

Try easing your own adaptation to postpartum parenting by formulating a plan such as the one below. Take one column at a time starting at the left. You might find it useful to complete your joint plan first, and then ask potential helpers to look over parts of it. Incidentally, do not be shy about asking for help; by asking, you are letting others know that you need them, trust them, respect them, and want to share an important event. Trust them to let you know if they cannot or do not want to help. Before you ask for help or accept offers of help, check with yourself and your partner to be sure that the help you ask for is really something you need and not something that will add to the stress of this time. Some individuals would be terrible to have around the house when a new baby arrives, but would do a wonderful job of supplying meals during that first week. Specify what you need from each helper. They will usually be happy to know that their effort is really needed.

In column I, jot down the needs you foresee during the period immediately following the birth of your baby (the first few weeks). Write down anything that comes to mind. Make as long a list as you can.

In column II, rank them in order of importance. Remember that this is a crisis time and relatively short-lived, so you might use this perspective to really zero in on the top ten needs you have.

In column III, check areas of conflict, including conflict between you and your partner, people on the job, relatives, doctor, etc.—and within yourselves. Try to describe these briefly, and in your responses, specify solutions to these conflicts as well as solutions which meet needs that are not in conflict.

In column IV, select some ways to meet your needs and resolve your conflicts during pregnancy, and in column V, decide how you will cope with these needs during the postpartum period.

Columns VI and VII are for recording who will do what, when, and where.

Jackie and Mac Adams' Postpartum Crisis Survival Plan (Condensed)

Needs	Rank	Conflicts	Solutions: Pregnancy	Postpartum
			Rest:	
Rest	3	X (Mac is tired of a tired wife)	1. Resign volunteer jobs 2. Plan to limit social life	1. Make daily rest plan and time together plan 2. Mac takes time off work to help
Lose weight	12			
			Breastfeeding	
Breastfeeding	2		1. Attend La Leche League mtgs. 2. Reading 3. Discuss with Mac and friends 4. Find supportive pediatrician 5. Nurse on delivery table 6. Arrange for rooming-in 7. Return home early from hospital 8. Start nipple toughening now	1. Nurse on demand 2. Continue La Leche Leag* 3. Stay in phone contact with LLL leader 4. Rest 5. Avoid others who don't approve 6. Don't offer bottles
Finish bathroom walls	14			
Clean house	10			
Sex	9	X		
			Time Alone:	
Time alone	5		1. Discover one thing I really love to do (both of us)	1. Alternate caring for baby away fro* 2. Trade sitting with other nursing couple*

| Implementation | |
Pregnancy	Postpartum
1. J: line up a household helper now 2. Resign volunteer jobs by eighth month 3. J/M: tell all who invite that acceptance contingent on no baby 4. J/M: organize friends and relations to provide food, diaper service, shopping, and to leave us alone during first weeks	1. J/M: plan first thing in morning 2. M: calls helper and handles directions, payment, etc. 3. M: See job
1. J: monthly meetings 2. J/M: read *Motherly Art of Breastfeeding.* Buy for reference 3. J/M: discuss hospital-related items with midwife. Repeat several times to remind her 4. J/M: do nipple toughening together nightly 5. Locate pediatrician as soon as possible. Ask at LLL meetings. Ask midwife. J/M see him together for consultation, eighth month	1. J: Line up meetings during pregnancy. M drives J and baby to and from meetings 2. J/M decide who is antibreastfeeding: M handles them 3. M reminds J of importance of rest and close contact with La Leche League leader
1. Discuss this together. Try to help each other discover favorite activities. Do it next weekend on trip to Berkshire Music Festival with wine and cheese	1. J/M: plan locations, decide what to do with baby together 2. J: during pregnancy, find an agreeable nursing couple through LLL

Needs	Rank	Conflicts	Solutions: Pregnancy	Postpartum
			Enjoy Baby:	
Enjoy baby	1	X (No one wants to take care of a grumpy baby)	1. Learn baby care and practice (Check to see if Sal and Jill will let us practice on Joshua)	1. Play with baby on mattress while changing diapers
Reading	11		2. Line up a postpartum class	2. Take baths in bathtub with baby (after umbilical cord heals)
Teach T.M.	13		3. Buy a Snugli	3. Share family bed
			4. Buy a huge foam mattress and put it on the floor in our bedroom plus covers, etc.	4. Take baby and J to fun places in Snugli
			5. Get lots of diapers and a new washing machine and dryer	5. J/M: discuss and agree on standards of care, so that M and J both feel comfortable caring for baby alone
			6. Ask for easy-to-put-on-and-take-off clothes	6. J: express some milk, and put it in the freezer in a bottle. Practice M feeding this to baby once in a while; so baby and M can stay together alone
			7. Build a swinging basket for baby, and put mountings in ceiling in kitchen, living room, and bedroom	

Implementation:

Pregnancy	Postpartum
1. Attend family-centered childbirth class together	1. M: changes diapers when he is home
2. J: call S & J and ask. J/M both practice (maybe take care of Joshua for an afternoon)	2. M: bathes baby when he is home at bath time
3. J/M: line up a postpartum class and Snugli through midwife, childbirth teacher, or La Leche League leader	3. J/M: plan to disagree a lot on what is good baby care. Try to be tolerant and see this as a time of learning a tough job under strain
4. M: buy mattress from Sears catalogue. J: order covers	
5. J/M: Read *Family Bed* in childbirth class library	
6. Buy washer/dryer and diapers eighth month, together	
7. J: make a list of gifts baby needs now and distribute to friends and relatives	
8. Get plans for swing from FAMILY, 155 W. 4th St., Fulton, NY 13069. Set it up eighth month	

Needs	Rank	Conflicts	Solutions: Pregnancy	Postpartum
			M-Feel Easy About Job:	
Feel easy about job	4	X (Jackie wants Mac home with her)	1. Discuss needs with Mr. P (boss)	1. Stay in touch with office daily
Cooking	6		2. Clear slate by working extra hours now	2. Work part-time for a while after first two or three days after birth
Shopping	7		3. Train others to take over key projects	3. Take some work home
Pay bills	8		4. Save up vacation time	4. Try hard to get enough sleep
			5. Work out an agreement in case an emergency happens and Mac must return to work What constitutes an emergency? What can M and J do to minimize the chances? To know ahead of time? To get back home fast? Who will substitute for M at home?	5. Stay open to Jackie about how I am feeling about work
			6. Decide whether this job is more antifatherhood than is right for you two	6. After 2 weeks, start working a short week
			7. Investigate how others at work and elsewhere have dealt with this	7. Be careful not to daydream; try to stay alert and *into* what I am doing at the time NO vague anxieties
				8. Use phone to do all possible work from home

Implementation:

Pregnancy	Postpartum
1. Set appointment with Mr. P for next week. Plan to meet casually several times on this. Let him know this is really important to me. Express feelings	1. Take work home only on weekends
	2. J: ask her to remind me—no daydreaming and no murder mysteries for first six weeks
2. Let him know all I am trying to do is to gain time and ease of mind so he appreciates this effort and does not just add more work. Ask him for ideas, have him review my plan (give it to him in writing, along with phone #, etc., so he can get in touch with me easily.) Put emergency plan in writing, too	3. J promises to be assertive about her need to have me around, but to understand my anxiety about being seen as a shirker by others at work
	4. Phone office 11 A.M. and 4 P.M. daily
	5. Jackie helps me recognize my anxieties by asking me how I am doing once in a while
3. Train secretary and Rick to handle my stuff duing this time. Have a trial run a month before due date. Work out a phone contact plan; what's worth calling about, phone dictation, what's an emergency, and so on. Make them feel included and try to work out a repayment plan with them	6. If Mr. P and the others cannot accept this, or I cannot feel relaxed with this, then J and I should seriously look at the idea of a new job, maybe even a new career, which allows more freedom to be a father and husband. Look at this question throughout but most carefully about 3 months after the birth
5. Make sure that Jackie knows what I have arranged with others	
6. Check with LLL (Jackie), childbirth class, midwife, and library for ideas on other solutions	

Information Directory

There has been an information explosion in recent years about pregnancy, birth, breastfeeding, and parenting. These organizations and publications are primary sources for further information as you plan your childbearing years.

Nutrition

Society for the Protection of the Unborn through Nutrition (SPUN)
17 N. Wabash Ave., Suite 603
Chicago, IL 60602
Telephone: (312) 332-2334
This agency counsels pregnant women nationwide about nutrition, provides speakers for parent and professional meetings, trains pregnancy nutrition counselors, evaluates research on malnutrition and developmental disabilities, publishes newsletters and materials for nutrition counseling.

Through the **Litigation Information Center,** they provide information about malpractice and liability suits in progress about incorrect pregnancy nutrition management, assist in locating expert witnesses, and refer prospective plaintiffs to attorneys interested in malnutrition litigation.

The New York office operates a **National Toxemia Hotline** for consultation about possible cases of metabolic toxemia: testing, obtaining medical records, hospital procedures, and medical management.
Telephone: (914) 271-6474

Childbirth

American Academy of Husband-Coached Childbirth (The Bradley Method)
P.O. Box 5224
Sherman Oaks, CA 91413
Telephone: (213) 788-6662
This organization was founded by Marge and Jay Hathaway in 1970 to promote the method of natural childbirth developed by Dr. Robert A. Bradley of Denver in 1947. AAHCC trains instructors and develops materials for use in childbirth education classes. They feature a strong nutrition

program, provide relaxation training for labor, stress avoidance of drugs, advocate father participation in pregnancy and birth, and provide effective consumer advocacy.

They also offer referrals to affiliated teachers nationwide.

American College of Home Obstetrics

664 N. Michigan Ave., Suite 610
Chicago, IL 60611
Telephone: (312) 642-7472

This is a society of physicians and others interested in setting standards for training home birth attendants, and they are also concerned with obtaining recognition of home obstetrics as a separate medical specialty.

American Foundation for Maternal and Child Health

30 Beekman Place
New York, NY 10022
Telephone: (212) 759-5510

They research the effects of obstetric management on maternal and infant outcome. They sponsor an annual conference reflecting the interdisciplinary approach to the problems of maternity care.

Association for Childbirth at Home, International (ACHI) National Headquarters

6840 Orangethorpe Ave., Suite E
Buena Park, CA 92060
Telephone: (213) 802-1020

Founded in 1972 by Tonya Brooks, this agency makes information about home birth available to expectant parents. ACHI also trains leaders of parent classes, offers advanced leader training for people attending births, holds conferences, and publishes a home birth manual tailored to those who cannot arrange medical assistance. They offer referrals to leaders nationwide.

Cooperative Childbirth Network

14 Truesdale Dr.
Croton-on-Hudson, NY 10520
Telephone: (914) 271-6474

The network develops resources for woman-centered childbearing. Their list of materials includes: Cooperative Childbirth course outlines, course slides and tapes, newsletter, instructor training seminars, and reprints for expectant women dealing with the women's health issues central to childbearing. Associates of the network are largely childbirth specialists with broad experience in a wide variety of birth methods and philosophies. Referrals available nationally.

National Association of Parents and Professionals for Safe Alternatives in Childbirth (NAPSAC)
National Headquarters
P.O. Box 267
Marble Hill, MO 63764
Telephone: (314) 238-2010

NAPSAC is dedicated to exploring, examining, and establishing family-centered childbirth programs in and out of hospitals. The goals of such programs are to meet the human needs of family members as well as to provide the safe aspects of medical science. In its role as a forum, facilitating communication and cooperation among parents, medical professionals, and childbirth educators, NAPSAC sponsors an annual conference on childbirth reform which has been endorsed and/or approved for educational credit by the professional organizations of nurses, midwives, obstetricians, family practitioners, osteopaths, and pediatricians. Conference proceedings are published each year as quality paperback books which are then used as references or texts in many medical, nursing, and public health schools. Through the **Institute for Childbirth and Family Research,** NAPSAC supports scientific investigation into alternatives in childbearing. Local groups exist in most parts of the country.

Institute for Childbirth and Family Research
2522 Dana St., Suite 201
Berkeley, CA 94704
Telephone: (415) 849-3665

FAMILY: Family-Centered Childbirth and Parenting
155 W. Fourth St.
Fulton, NY 13069
Telephone: (315) 598-7868

Jane and Jim Pittenger originated FAMILY in 1975 to educate expectant parents about childbearing as part of a marital relationship. FAMILY trains couples who wish to teach childbirth classes together. They offer referrals to affiliated teaching couples in New York, Connecticut, and New Jersey.

Breastfeeding

La Leche League International
9616 Minneapolis Ave.
Franklin Park, IL 60131
Telephone: (312) 455-7730

This is a worldwide organization dedicated to good mothering through breastfeeding. They publish pamphlets, bulletins, newsletters, and the manual, *The Womanly Art of Breastfeeding*. They train leaders of groups which meet in most communities to assist women who want to breast-feed. They maintain a 24-hour individual counseling service by telephone and can refer questions about special nursing situations to a medical advisory board.

Human Lactation Center (Research)
666 Sturges Highway
Westport, CT 06880

This center conducts research on breastfeeding from cultural, nutritional, and developmental viewpoints. They also publish the *Lactation Quarterly*.

Midwifery

American College of Nurse-Midwives
1000 Vermont Ave. NW
Washington, DC 20005
Telephone: (202) 347-5445

The professional organization for certified nurse-midwives in the United States, it was founded in 1929 and offers guidelines and accreditation for midwifery educational programs in the United States.

International Confederation of Midwives

Established in 1922 to advance the profession of midwifery through greater international cooperation, the ICM membership consists of national groups of midwives. The American representative is: Dorothea Lang, C.N.M., M.P.H., Director of

Midwifery Services, MIC Project, NYC Department of Health, 377 Broadway, New York, NY 10013.
Telephone: (212) 966-3828

National Midwives Association
1119 E. San Antonio Ave.
El Paso, TX 79901
Telephone: (915) 533-8142
  This organization publishes a newsletter for practicing midwives and sponsors conferences and workshops for new and experienced midwives.

Maternity Center Association
48 E. Ninety-second St.
New York, NY 10028
Telephone: (212) 369-7300
  This is a pioneering midwife-staffed maternity service that originated the concept of prenatal care and childbirth education in the United States. They opened an out-of-hospital birth center in 1975 where families come for comprehensive care for the childbearing years. They publish materials about childbearing and their current operations, philosophy, and practice.

Women's Health

Feminist Women's Health Centers
1112 Crenshaw Blvd.
Los Angeles, CA 90019
Telephone: (213) 936-6293
  Self-help materials are available from this group by mail. They offer referrals to other health clinics run by women across the country and to new pregnancy groups affiliated with MOTHER.

Health Right
175 Fifth Ave.
New York, NY 10010
Telephone: (212) 674-3660
  This society publishes a newsletter of the women's health movement and other pamphlets and position papers on a wide variety of issues relating to women's health. They give courses and workshops on health and the politics of the health care system.

Other Resources

ACHI Supplies Center
R.D. 9 Fair St.
Carmel, NY 10512
Telephone: (914) 225-7763

A mail-order service for books, slides, and teaching aids for childbirth, midwifery, breastfeeding, and child rearing. Their catalog is sent free of charge.

ICEA Supplies Center
P.O. Box 70258
Seattle, WA 98107
Telephone: (206) 789-4444

This organization supplies books by mail on a wide variety of subjects relating to the childbearing years. They publish *Bookmarks Quarterly*, a review of new books in the field.

National Foundation of the March of Dimes
Genetic Counseling Centers
1275 Mamaroneck Ave.
White Plains, NY 10605
Telephone: (914) 428-7100

They offer a referral service to genetic counseling centers around the world.

American Fertility Society
1608 Thirteenth Ave. S
Suite 101
Birmingham, AL 35205
Telephone: (205) 933-7222

Planned Parenthood-World Population
810 Seventh Ave.
New York, NY 10019
Telephone: (212) 541-7800

Index

Page numbers in italics indicate illustrations.